Re-Visioning Spirit:
A Brief Introduction To Thumotics

Your Spirit, Your Life Series
Book 1
Second Edition

Mark W. Neville, MDiv

Copyright © 2016, 2019 Mark W Neville

Second Edition

All rights reserved.

ISBN: 10:1537003038
ISBN: 13:9781537003030

DEDICATION

To all the living.

*"It is the function of art to renew our perception.
What we are familiar with we cease to see.
The writer shakes up the familiar scene, and, as if by magic,
we see a new meaning in it."
Anais Nin*

CONTENTS

	Acknowledgments	i
1	Thumotics and Monocrats	1
2	Wonder!	9
3	What is Spirit?	13
4	Spiritual Language	27
5	Loving Care of Spirit	35
6	Spiritual Knowledge	43
7	Spiritual Healing	62
8	Spirituality	72
9	Spiritual Community	81
	Afterword	88
	For Further Reading	91
	Thumotic Lexicon	93
	About the Author	103

ACKNOWLEDGMENTS

This book exists only by
the inspiration of
Homer and his devotees,
Friedrich Nietzsche, Seth Godin, Stephen Crites,
my hospice patients and their family members,
my former hospice colleagues, my private clients,
and most important of all, Lisa, the love of my life.
Without her I could not breathe.

From my heart to yours,
deep gratitude and love.

Mark W. Neville

1 THUMOTICS AND MONOCRATS

A strong spirit transcends rules- Prince

Purpose of This Book

The purpose of this book is to disturb and inspire you. It is about spirit, but not as you might see it now. If you are like most Westerners, you see spirit in materialistic, religious, metaphysical, or psychological terms. Ironically, if you are among the materialists who dismiss the existence of spirit, you probably share the same view of spirit as the majority of Westerners. You just deny its existence.

Audience

This book is not for everyone. It is for the brave few willing to leap first into a new way of seeing spirit, themselves, and the world in which we live. It is not for those who are comfortable under the rule of a monocrat of their mind, compliantly accepting their ruler's answers as their own, and no longer able to wonder. It is for the few, free and open-minded enough to consider Thumotics.

Thumotics Defined

Thumotics is a word derived from the Ancient Greek word for spirit, *thumos*. It is an umbrella term that covers a number of theoretical and practical domains based on a re-visioning of spirit. It includes a clear definition of spirit as well as a new science, therapy, and spirituality of spirit. It begins with being wondered by life.

Overview of Chapters

Socrates once said, "Wonder is the beginning of wisdom." This chapter introduces Thumotics and the monocrats of our minds that might prevent us from seeing spirit in a new way.

Chapter Two invites you to wonder anew at the mere fact that we are alive rather than not. It encourages you to wonder about questions inspired by the mere fact of being alive.

Chapter Three presents the re-visioning of spirit in terms of the Ancient Greek word for spirit: *thumos*. Re-visioning spirit in terms of *thumos* demands that we also revise what we mean by the words "spirited", "spiritual", "spirituality", and everything related to these words. Re-visioning spirit in terms of *thumos* is the heart of this book. Everything else is commentary.

Chapters Four through Nine spin out the implications of re-visioning spirit in terms of *thumos*. They revision-

Our language about spirit

Spiritual care as philothumy, befriending spirit

Spiritual knowledge as thumology, the scientific study of spirit

Spiritual healing as thumotherapy, the healing of spirit based on philothumy and thumology

Spirituality as the quality of having spirit

Spiritual community as a group united by sharing a common characteristic, interest, or practice related to spirit.

The Afterword invites the reader to imagine and help realize a future inspired by the re-visioning of spirit introduced in this book. A list of books for further reading and a lexicon of Thumotics finish the book.

The Re-Visioning Spirit Series

This brief introduction to Thumotics is the first in a series called *Your Spirit, Your Life*. The subjects introduced in this book will be expanded into a series of books which include the following titles:

Your Little Book of Spiritual Knowledge: A New Holistic View

Affirmations of Life

Your Life: An Owner's Manual

Spiritual Sayings for Earthlings

Life Zones: How to Make Your Way to a Better Place in Life

Your Little Book of Spiritual Practices

Life Therapy: An Phenomenal Approach to Life

Re-Visioning Theologia

Barriers to Re-Visioning Spirit: Monocrats of Our Minds

Barriers stand between where we are now as Westerners and the re-visioning of spirit presented in this brief introduction. The barriers are our loyalties to monocrats of our mind who dictate *how* we know, *what* we know, and what we *value*. The monocrats of *how* we know include rationalism, empiricism, and religiosity.

Monocrats of *How* We Know

Rationalism is extreme loyalty to reason. It is the belief that by reason alone we know what is true. Rene Descartes expressed this belief with profound influence on Western culture when he said "I think, therefore I am."

Empiricism is extreme loyalty to sense perception. It is the belief that by sense perception alone we know what is true. Emmanuel Kant expressed this belief with profound influence on Western culture when he said, " All our knowledge begins with the senses."

Religiosity is extreme loyalty to religion. It is the belief that by faith alone in the doctrines of a religion we know what is true. This loyalty was expressed with profound influence on Western culture by Augustine, the bishop of Hippo, when he said, "Believe that you may understand."

If reason, sense perception, or religion rules as a monocrat of your mind, Thumotics might disturb you. These monocrats rule out other ways of knowing. To understand Thumotics, you will have to betray the one who now rules *how* you gain knowledge. Such treason might be too disturbing for you.

Monocrats of *What* We Know

The monocrats of *what* we know include *idealism, realism, materialism, dualism, and psychologism*. *Idealism* is extreme loyalty to the ideas in our minds. It is the belief that we know only ideas in our mind. Idealism dictates that if things exist apart from us, we do not know them as they are. We only know our ideas of them. We do not know the tree we see. We only know the idea of the tree in our mind. Idealists cannot know spirit. They can only know the idea of spirit.

Realism, on the other hand, is extreme loyalty to the correspondence between what we know and our knowledge of it. It is the belief that what we perceive with our five physical senses matches exactly what exists independently of our perceptions. What we know is the real thing itself. The tree we see really is as we see it. Realists tend to reject the existence of spirit because they cannot know what they cannot see.

Materialism is extreme loyalty to matter - regardless of whether matter is wave, particle, or both. It is the belief that what we know is matter alone. All is matter. Materialists either reject the existence of spirit or reduce it to physical matter. They believe that if spirit exists at all, it is best explained in terms of physics.

Dualism, on the other hand, is extreme loyalty to the dualism of the physical versus the "spiritual." It is the belief that reality consists of two different principles: the physical known by sense perception and the "spiritual" known by faith (or mental known by introspection). They believe that what we know about the physical world are facts and we only have beliefs or opinions about the "spiritual" world. Therefore, we should all agree on the facts, but everyone is free to have their own private beliefs and opinions about the "spiritual" world. For Dualists, whether or not spirit exists and how it is defined are matters of private belief and opinion, not matters of fact and public concern.

Psychologism is a child of Dualism. It is extreme loyalty to the mind-body duality. It is Dualism at the human level. It is the belief that what we know about humans is that we consist of two principles that influence each other: mind and body. Psychologism, if it acknowledges the existence of spirit at all, attributes no existence of spirit apart from mind. In psychologism, spirit is conflated with mind.

Idealism, Realism, Materialism, Dualism, and *Psychologism* are barriers to re-visioning spirit. Thumotics challenges these monocratic loyalties of mind. To comprehend Thumotics, you will have to dethrone the monocrat that dictates *what* you know. Such rebellion might be too disturbing for you.

Monocrats of What We *Value*

The third and last set of monocrats that hinder us from re-visioning spirit have to do with what we *value*. They include *humanism, individualism, hedonism,* and *metaphysicalism*.

Humanism is extreme loyalty to Human Being. Humanists value human beings above all others, animate and inanimate, physical, and spiritual. They believe humans are superior to and rightly dominate all others on Earth. Even if they are atheists, they believe in some sense these words from the book of Genesis, "And God blessed them [the humans], and God said unto them, 'Be fruitful, and multiply, and replenish the earth, and subdue it: and have dominion over the fish of the sea, and over the fowl of the air, and over every living thing that moveth upon the earth.'" Humanists devalue the spirit of all but human beings.

Individualism is extreme loyalty to the Individual. Individualists value individual human beings above society or any other kind of group. They believe in the ultimate value of individual freedom. "Give me liberty or give me death!" they cry with Patrick Henry. Individualists tend to devalue, if not ignore, the importance of relationships and the spirit of groups.

Hedonism is extreme loyalty to Self-Gratification. It values individual self-gratification above all else. Hedonists share the faith of King Solomon that the ultimate value is to "Eat, drink, and be merry!" They fail to acknowledge the life-denying impact they have on their own spirit and that of others.

Metaphysicalism is extreme loyalty to the Spiritual. It values the "spiritual" side of the physical versus spiritual duality. Metaphysicalists value being "spiritual". They believe that the less this-worldly and more other-worldly we are, the more "spiritual" we are. The more "spiritual" we are, the better we are. They believe we are just visitors, passing through this world, on our way to our true home in heaven or some other metaphysical realm. They fail to see spirit in this world and deny the value of both this world and spirit in it.

Liberation

If you feel comfortable and safe ruled by a monocrat of your mind, this book is probably not for you. If you read this far, thank you.

If you are ruled by a monocrat of your mind and long to be free, you can be. But it is not easy. It requires physical, mental, and emotional labor. It requires rebellion. You must overthrow the monocrat of your mind and adopt self-rule. Become your own monocrat. Rule yourself rather than be ruled by another.

Liberating yourself will cost you. You might pay the price by grieving the loss of relationships with family members and friends who are dear to you. You will definitely pay the price of dying to your current way of life and rising up to live into a new way.

Once you free yourself, you will have some distance between you and your former as well as the other monocrats of the mind. Each monocrat has some truth and value. The distance allows you to take from each what serves you and drop the rest.

Once free, you can also affirm in a new way your own life as well as the lives of all others. You might also see the value of Thumotics and the problems it addresses.

Problems Addressed by Thumotics

Thumotics addresses four significant problems that challenge many Westerners today. It addresses the—

- Lack of a general consensus on the meaning of the word "spirit" and all words related to it, such as aspire, conspire, dispirit, expire, inspire, respire, spire, spirited, spiritual, spirituality, and transpire

- Privatization of spirit and consequential lack of a coherent public conversation about spirit and everything related to it

- Metaphysicalism and religiosity that devalue life in this world and rationalize human disregard for this world (anthropocentrism, racism, sexism, waste, pollution, depletion, extinction, domination, violence, war, and poverty) while exalting a future life in a so-called spiritual world.

- Scientism that reduces the only knowledge of value to what fits in the overlapping boxes of empiricism, rationalism, and materialism

Six Characteristics of Thumotics

Thumotics addresses the problems identified above with six characteristics regarding its re-visioning of spirit. In Thumotics matters of spirit are—

1. Clearly-defined rather than vague and varying
2. Western-rooted rather than Eastward turning
3. Nature-based rather than otherworldly-based
4. Holistically-known rather than known only by reason, sense perception, or faith
5. Spirit-focused rather than religion- or psychology-focused
6. Life-affirming rather than life-denying

Vision of Thumotics

Thumotics does present a vision: a world in which more of us value that we are alive rather than not and live more life-affirming lives. The life-affirming lives envisioned in this book are human lives characterized by-

Thauma (Wonder): Being open to being wondered by the fact that we are alive rather than not and to the curiosity it inspires

Aidos (Humility): Living well-grounded, close-to-Earth lives

Holognosis (Holistic knowing): Drawing on all sources of knowledge

Harmonia (Harmony, concord): Living in tune with ourselves as unique individuals in unique groups and all other unique individuals and groups.

Chapter Two is about *thauma* (wonder). If you have read this far, thank you. Perhaps this book is for you. Please, read on.

2 WONDER!

Once we believe in ourselves, we can risk curiosity, wonder, spontaneous delight, or any experience that reveals the human spirit. - e. e. cummings

Everyday Wondering

Every day we wonder about everyday things: what to wear, what to eat, what to do. If we are privileged to have a computer and internet access, we might also wonder about answers to questions a quick internet search away: the weather forecast, directions to our destination, information about a topic of current interest, the possible side effects of a medication we are taking. But not all of our questions have answers an internet search away.

More Serious Wondering

Sometimes we wonder about more serious questions: what will I do with my life, where can I get a job, what is wrong with me, where will I get the medical care I need, how will I pay for it, will I survive?

We also wonder about things other than ourselves- our family, lover, friends, co-workers, neighbors, business, those in need, our country, the world.

Being Wondered

There are also times when we are wondered. Something marvels us, grabs our whole being, and stops us: a blazing sunset, shooting star, brilliant rainbow, majestic tree, mesmerizing song, stunning painting, extraordinary athletic feat, kind act of another person, or anything that wows us. When we are wondered we feel marveled, stop, look, and stand in silent rapture or utter an involuntary "Wow!", "Ahhh...", "That's amazing!" or "Look at that!"

Being wondered fills us. Our fullness overflows, and we have to tell others about it. Doing so prolongs our feeling of being wondered and spreads it to others.

Being wondered also inspires curiosity. It draws us in for a closer look. Questions arise: "What is it?" "How did that happen?", "Why did that happen?", "What did it mean?"

Be Wondered Anew

This book is an invitation to being wondered anew by something basic. We easily take it as granted until it is threatened or taken away. We do not physically see, hear, touch, taste, or smell it, but we experience it every day. It is a fact, not just an idea or religious belief. We know first-hand it is real.

Be wondered by this: You are alive.

You are alive with others.

Wonder of wonders! You are alive! We are alive rather than not!

Being alive is not something to take as granted. Once you were not alive. You were conceived, gestated, and born. Now you are alive and have developed to the point of reading this book. The moment will come when you die. No one knows when that moment will come. However, right now, wonder of wonders, you are alive rather than not.

Be Curious

Socrates said, "Wonder is the beginning of wisdom."

Let the wonder of being alive marvel you, draw you in, and inspire questions that nourish your wisdom:

Why Life?

Why is there life rather than not?

Why are you among the living at this time rather than not?

Why are we alive together?

What is Life?

What does it mean to be alive?

What is the difference between being alive and not?

What makes you alive rather than not?

The Beginning, Sustaining, and Purpose of Life?

Did life have a beginning? If so, when and how?

What sustains life? What hinders it?

Why sex? Why the intimacy between sex and life?

What drives us to keep living and reproducing?

Does being alive have a purpose? If so, how do we know? What is it?

Is there a best way to live? If so, what is it?

The End of Life and Afterlife?

What happens when we die? What is death?

Will all life end? If so, when? How?

Is there life after death?

Life, sex, and death. These are the three great wonders of life.

This brief introduction to Thumotics revels in these great wonders and the questions they inspire.

The next chapter is about what makes us alive rather than not.

3 WHAT IS SPIRIT?

*...the first instinct of spirituality,
the spirit's instinct for self-preservation. - Friedrich Nietzsche*

Wonder of wonders! You are alive! We are alive together!

What does it mean to be alive? What is the difference between being alive and not? What makes us alive rather than not?

This chapter moves from being *wondered by* the fact of being alive to *wondering about* being alive rather than not. It is about being inspired with curiosity, drawing near, allowing questions to arise, living with those questions and finding out where they lead. This chapter is the heart of this brief introduction and Thumotics as a whole. It begins with the story of what inspired me to wonder about spirit. It happened when I was a clinical director of a nationally recognized hospice organization.

What Inspired Me to Wonder About Spirit

I began my career in hospice in 2005 as a spiritual care professional caring for hospice patients and their family members. Most of the hospice patients I cared for cared about life. They weren't dying. They were living and committed to living as well as they could for however much time they had left. They cared about the quality of their life more than its length, the life in their days more than the days in their life. They were focused on what mattered most to them as they lived out the end of their life. I learned a lot about life and living from my hospice patients.

In 2007, I became the clinical coordinator of the bereavement and music therapy teams. My bereaved clients also taught me a lot about life and living.

Then I became the clinical director of the hospice team that cared for patients in assisted living communities as well as the spiritual care, bereavement, and music therapy teams. Because I was also trained in complementary and alternative therapies, I started and directed the complementary and alternative medicine program. It fit beautifully into the holistic approach of hospice care.

During my time as a spiritual care professional and clinical director, I was asked to teach new employees (physicians, nurses, nurse assistants, social workers, and managers) about spiritual care, bereavement, and complementary and alternative medicine. I did this for several years. During the same time, I also taught palliative care physicians and other palliative care professionals from all over the United States about spiritual care, bereavement, and complementary and alternative medicine.

To teach others, I had to think deeper about and do research on the subjects. Spiritual care was the most challenging. I was both wondered by and wondered about spiritual care. The questions arose: What is spiritual care? What do the words "spiritual" and "care" mean? What do those who provide spiritual care actually do?

On Caring

I learned the most about what it means to care by observing and listening to my patients and families. They taught me how best to care for them. I also learned about caring from the hospice physicians, nurses, social workers, music therapists, and chaplains with whom I worked. I learned from how they cared for their patients and families. I also learned a lot from Milton Meyeroff's book, *On Caring*.

On Spirit

Answering the questions about spiritual care were far more challenging. What is "spiritual care"? What does the word "spiritual" mean? A dictionary said that "spiritual" meant "of, about, or related to spirit." This raised the question, "What is spirit?" From where did we get the word? What does it mean? The definition that resonated with me was "that which makes alive."

The more I studied spirit, the more I was wondered by the mere fact of being alive. Wonder of wonders! I am alive rather than not! You are alive rather than not! Everything living is alive rather than not!

Holistic and Integrative Health

Because hospice care is holistic and the hospice I was with was open to integrative medicine, I regularly attended the annual Mountain Area Health Education Center (MAHEC) integrative health conference in Asheville, North Carolina. In 2009, Dr. Andrew Weil, M.D. was the keynote speaker. Dr. Larry Dossey, M.D. and Dr. Barbara Dossey, PhD, R.N were featured speakers. Other well-known speakers gave presentations and demonstrations in breakout sessions. Every speaker talked about both holistic and integrative health care. They all were committed to caring for the whole person-body, mind, and spirit- and integrating Western and Eastern medicine to do so.

Only physicians, nurses, and providers of specific therapies gave presentations. No one specializing in mental/behavioral health or spiritual care spoke. In fact, based on a show of hands from the audience, I was the only professional spiritual care provider among the approximately five hundred participants.

"Spirituality"

The speakers talked mostly about care of the body. They also talked about psycho-social care and the mind-body connection. Without exception, if and when they talked about spiritual care, they talked about it last, gave it the least time, and spoke about it terms of spirituality rather than care of the person's spirit.

If they defined spirituality, it was admittedly their own personal definition and expressed their own personal beliefs and practices. They generally spoke of spirituality in existential terms as being about what each individual patient found meaningful and gave them a sense of self-transcendence.

In their view, religious beliefs and practices were meaningful for some. For others, family, love, nature, their personal eclectic belief system, meditation, music, helping others, reading, hiking, gardening, bird watching, having sex, enjoying food and drink, sports, travel, or other activities were meaningful. Whatever was personally meaningful and gave a sense of transcendence was considered their spirituality.

"Anyone Can Do Spiritual Care"

The speakers further stated either directly or indirectly, that anyone could provide spiritual care; that is, anyone could care about what a patient found meaningful. It was relatively simple: listen, reflect back what you heard, pray with the patient if the patient asks and you are comfortable with it, and call for a chaplain if a longer prayer is needed or there are religious needs that only clergy can address.

My Inspiration: An Insight

During Dr. Larry Dossey's plenary presentation on the mind-body connection, my inspiration came. It flashed in my mind with brilliant clarity as a full-blown, multi-faceted, whole and integrated insight. Prior to this insight, I shared the status quo view of spirituality described above. After this insight everything changed. Below are the facets of the insight. You can verify for yourself whether they are accurate or not.

- In healthcare, if spiritual care is provided, it is care for patients' spirituality and/or religious beliefs rather than their spirit. Spiritual care is assumed to be care of a patient's spirit. It is not.

- Generally, Western medicine, based on Western science, denies the existence of spirit. At best, it ignores it. At worst, it harms it.

- In holistic and integrative medicine, we often *say* we care for the whole person: body, mind, and spirit. What we actually *do* is care for body, mind, and spirituality.

- We have in healthcare a clear general consensus about what the words "body" and "mind" refer to. We ignore spirit and have no clear general consensus about what the words "spirit", "spiritual", and "spirituality" refer to. However, we often speak as if everyone shares a common understanding of what these words mean.

- "Spiritual care" is often a synonym (or euphemism) for religious care or existential counseling. It is often, in theory and practice, supporting what one finds meaningful and/or addressing religious needs. It is about caring for a person's spirituality, not a person's spirit.

- In verbal and written communication in healthcare, "spiritual" and "spirituality" are usually undefined, associated with religion or psychology, used to refer to something metaphysical or psychological, assigned to the category of personal opinion and belief rather than fact, and are sometimes used for emotional effect; that is, to give a "woo" factor as in "spiritual person", "spiritual belief", "spiritual experience", or "spiritual practice".

- We have well-developed sciences for the study of both the human body and mind. We have no scientific study of the human spirit. We cannot have such a science until we agree that spirit exists and have a general consensus on what spirit is.

- We have a general consensus on the difference between a healthy and unhealthy body and mind and have science-based therapies for both. We have no general consensus on the difference between a healthy and unhealthy spirit and have no science-based therapies for the ill or injured spirit. We cannot have a science-based therapy of spirit until we have a general consensus on what the human spirit is and scientific study devoted to it.

- The physicians, nurses, social workers, counselors, chaplains, and other healthcare professionals providing spiritual care often do so from their own personal understanding of what spirituality and spiritual care are.

- We require licensure of physicians, nurses, massage therapists, chiropractors, psychotherapists, and mental/behavioral health counselors. We do not require licensure of chaplains and other spiritual care professionals.

- Board-certified chaplains, believed by many to be the gold standard of spiritual care professionals, are primarily trained to address the religious needs of individuals of the chaplain's own religion. They are usually, not always, formally educated in their own religion, ordained or otherwise authorized for ministry by the authorities of their own religion, endorsed for ministry by the authorities of their own religion, and receive Clinical

Pastoral Education in which they are trained in existential psychology, counseling skills, and how to function in a clinical setting.

- In other words, we do not have professionals providing care for the human spirit. We have religious professionals providing care for religious needs and existential issues and concerns. Since they often address religious needs of clients of faiths different from their own, their religious care is at best a referral to officials of the client's religion. Perhaps too often chaplains address the needs of those with different faiths on their own, generically. Worst of all, chaplains attempt to convert their clients to their own faith. Since they are not well-trained in existential psychology, their existential counseling is often, at best, second rate.

Health Care: A Reflection of Society

Our healthcare industry is a reflection of our society and Western civilization at this time. We have problems with spirit in health care because we have problems with spirit in our society and Western civilization in general. We have no clear general consensus on the existence or definition of "spirit". Therefore, we have no general consensus on clear definitions of "spiritual" or "spirituality".

Our public discourse about spirit, spiritual, and spirituality is at best expressing our individual personal beliefs. We can believe anything we want about spirit, including that it does not exist. Likewise, we can believe anything we want about "spiritual" and "spirituality."

Imagine having no general consensus on what the words "body" and "mind" refer to. Imagine us all using those words to refer to whatever we individually wanted. We would have no scientific study of body or mind just as we now have no scientific study of spirit.

Since we have no scientific study and knowledge of what a healthy or unhealthy spirit is, we have no therapeutic care of ill and injured spirits. We therefore have no well-trained, licensed professionals who care for and nurture healthy spirits and heal ill and injured spirits when needed.

Wondering About "Spirit," "Spiritual," and "Spirituality"

The insight I had at the conference inspired questions that compelled me to wonder more deeply about spirit, what is spiritual, and what spirituality is.

We have a general consensus about what "body" and "mind" refer to. We have sciences devoted to them. We understand illnesses and injuries of both and have therapies for both provided by licensed professionals. What happened with spirit in our practice of medicine? What happened with spirit in Western civilization?

What does "spirit" mean? To what does it refer? What is it? To what do the words "spiritual" and "spirituality" refer? Can we reach a general consensus on the meaning of these words?

How might it look to have sciences devoted to the study of spirit? What might illnesses and injuries of spirit look like? What might therapies for healing an ill or injured spirit be? What could it look like to have licensed professional providers of care of spirit? What might their training need to be? I share what I discovered below.

What I Discovered

Before I share what I discovered about spirit, I encourage you to do your own wondering about spirit. Begin with yourself. How do you define the word "spirit"? What do the words "spiritual" and "spirituality" mean to you?

Look up the word "spirit" in various dictionaries. Do an internet search and read the results. Watch for the word in everything you read. What do the writers mean when they use the word "spirit"? Do the same with the words "spiritual" and "spirituality."

Listen for the words "spirit," "spiritual," and "spirituality" in spoken conversations and songs. When you have the opportunity, be politely curious and ask what the speaker means. Have a conversation. See what you learn.

Perhaps you will find something different or in addition to what I discovered. Here is an overview of what I discovered about the word "spirit":

Currently, our word "spirit" has a wide range of meaning. We use it without precision to refer to many different things. The following list is suggestive rather than exhaustive of what we use "spirit" to refer to-

- Part of a human that survives death: the spirit of a dead person, ghost

- A supernatural, non-physical being, like a nature spirit or angel.

- A malevolent, supernatural, non-physical being or energy that can enter and possess human beings: an evil spirit, devil, or demon.

- A universal, omnipresent, omnipotent, omniscient divine being, as in God, Great Spirit, or Holy Spirit

- A characteristic or attribute: "The spirit of the times."

- Loyalty to or enthusiasm for, as in team spirit: "Where's your team spirit?"

- The sense of a group acting as one: esprit de corps.

- The non-physical part of a human being and seat of the character, reason, and emotions; the mind or soul

- The part of a human being that survives death, synonymous with soul. "Her spirit lives on."

- A mood: "The sunny weather lifted our spirits."

- The real intention or meaning: "Follow the spirit and not just the letter of the law."

- Distilled liquor like whiskey, rum, or vodka: "No spirits are served here."

- Being energetic: "The horse has lots of spirit."

- Doing something with the desired attitude: "That's the spirit!"

- A continuing influence, legacy. "Her spirit still guides us even though she is not with us."

- What makes something alive rather than not. "His spirit is gone. He's dead."

Like the word "spirit" the words "spiritual" and "spirituality" also have wide ranges of meaning. "Spiritual" can be a synonym for religious, as in "spiritual beliefs" and "spiritual practices." It can refer to something metaphysical or supernatural, as in "a spiritual being." When used of a person, as in "spiritual person," it can refer to that person being more interested in religious, supernatural, or metaphysical things than physical, earthly things. "Spiritual" can refer to a type of religious song.

My conclusion is that many, because they do not like "religion", use "spirituality" to refer to their own personal eclectic religious beliefs.

How Did We Get Here?

How did we Westerners get to this place where we assigned the meaning of "spirit," "spiritual," and "spirituality" to personal, private belief and opinion? How did we get to this place where we lack a general consensus on what the words mean? How did we accept having no scientific study of spirit, no scientifically informed therapies for wounded and broken spirits, and no clear relationship of "spiritual" and "spirituality" with "spirit"?

Does our plethora of personal, private opinions and beliefs about what spirit is, what is spiritual, and what spirituality is serve us well? Does the opinion and belief that everyone has the freedom and right to believe whatever they want about what spirit is, what is spiritual, and what spirituality is serve us well? Would it serve us well if we all used the words "body" and "mind" to refer to whatever we wanted?

Could our plethora of opinions and beliefs, our lack a general consensus, be symptomatic of a deeper problem? Could it be symptomatic of problems related to our spirit? Spiritual problems? Problems with spirituality? I think so. I believe we Westerners have serious spiritual problems.

Digging Deeper

After researching how we currently use the words "spirit," "spiritual," and "spirituality" I dug deeper. I wondered about the origin of the word "spirit"? Where did it come from? To what did it refer in the past? Have we Westerners had a general consensus in the past about what spirit is?

It is not within the scope of this brief introduction to tell the whole story of the English, Germanic, Latin, and Greek words and concepts related to spirit. However, it is within the scope of this brief introduction to introduce the words and concepts relevant to Thumotics. Let's begin with Homer.

The *Iliad* and the *Odyssey* attributed to Homer are the oldest European literary works to survive intact and the twin foundation blocks of Western civilization. Ancient Greece, inspired by Homer's epics, is the mother and ongoing mentor of Western civilization. Is there a better place to begin a historical study of the concept of spirit in Western civilization? Thumotics is based on *thumos,* the Homeric word for spirit in the *Iliad* and the *Odyssey*.

The word *thumos* occurs over seven hundred times in Homer's epics. It refers to a very rich and complex human experience. It is associated with breath and wind, fumes, and refers to the life-breath, being alive, and liveliness. It is that which makes alive. It animates not only humans but the earth, mountains, valleys, springs, rivers, lakes, seas, plants (especially trees), animals, as well as goddesses and gods and other invisible beings.

Thumos is closely associated with *pneuma* and *psyche* but is not the same. *Thumos* is either present or not. It also varies in quantity and quality. When *thumos* leaves and returns, we call it fainting. When *thumos* leaves and does not return, we are dead. Unlike the *psyche* of humans, which remains after death and goes to Hades, the realm of the dead, *thumos* does not continue after death. It dissipates into the wind.

Thumos is quasi-physical, between physical and non-physical, not a physical organ but physically felt and closely associated with "heart." It is located in the center of our chest, between our breasts and behind our breast bone. It is also associated with our lungs. However, it also fills our whole being.

It, rather than our *psyche*, is the seat of all our emotions. We can feel in ourselves and others the variance of its quantity. The variance of its quantity is the variance of liveliness. In modern English, we speak of high and low spirits in reference to ourselves and others.

We can also feel in ourselves and others the variance of its quality. The variance of its quality we often refer to as spiritedness, character traits, emotions, and moods: He is mean-spirited. She has such a loving spirit. His spirit fills the room. Let's do something to lift her spirit.

Thumos also has a cognitive function. Consciousness is associated with *thumos*. We know things about ourselves and others in our *thumos*. We can deliberate with our *thumos*. We can argue with it and agree or disagree. We can act in accord or discord with our *thumos*. Our *thumos* can overwhelm our other physical and mental functions and compel our actions.

Thumos is associated with our thymus gland because of the gland's location behind our breast bone. It is also associated with the herb thyme both because of the similarities of shape between the thymus gland and thyme leaf and because thyme has a noticeable odor. *Thumos* is noticeable like the odor of thyme. Interestingly, thyme has a stimulating and strengthening effect. Greek warriors carried it with them into battle.

Our English word "spirit" came from the Latin word "spiritus." "Spiritus" meant "breath, wind, life, or that which makes alive." It is the root of many English words still in common use today: aspire, conspire, dispirit, expire, inspire, respirate, and transpire.

"Spiritus" superseded "anima" which meant the same thing. It is the root of "animal" and "animate." The Latin "animus" is a related word with the additional connotations of "intellect," "passion," and "wrath." It is the root of "animosity."

Scholars of Homer agree that *thumos* is best translated into English by the words "spirit," "spiritedness," and "heart." Here are some quotes from leading authorities on *thumos* in Homer:

"The etymology of *thumos* tells us that its basic meaning is breath, and specifically the breath of life. Hence, *thumos*, just like Homeric *psyche*, is breathed out when one dies...*Thumos*, I here propose, stands for the Homeric soul, and it should be translated by "spirit." A.A. Long, *Greek Models of Mind and Self*, p. 35.

"*Thumos* is known to us in English from the herb thyme which exudes a strong odor. "Fume" is a cognate in Latin...Thus the original meaning is 'breath' (of life), exhalation, ebullition, smoke, vapor. 'Spirit' which comes from the word for breath in Latin, *spiritus*, is a good translation for *thumos*. In Homeric epics it is often used for the vital principle, breathing life...But there is another sense, that of 'fuming,' of tempestuously roused spirit and of desire, appetite, and finally even friendliness...For this second set of meanings, "spiritedness" is probably the better term." Eva Brann, *Feeling Our Feelings: What Philosophers Think and People Know*, p. 23.

For more detailed information about Homeric *thumos*, see the books listed in *For Further Reading* on page ninety-one.

Wondering Whether or not Spirit Exists?

When we define spirit in terms of Homeric *thumos*, the question of whether or not spirit exists is easily answered. It is the same as asking if life exists. Yes, just as life exists, spirit exists. Spirit and life co-exist. Where there is life, there is spirit. Where there is spirit, there is life. They exist as one.

Just as life is inseparable from time and is chronological, so is spirit. We experience and express life as a narrative with a beginning, middle, and end; so it is with spirit. The story of a life is the story of a spirit. Spirit transpires as a narrative. Life and spirit expire together. They co-terminate. No life, no spirit. No spirit, no life.

Is spirit something separate from life? No, spirit is that which makes alive. What is the nature of spirit? That is the same as asking, "What is the nature of life?"

Life is an organic, unfolding story. So is our spirit. Just as our life is a narrative, so is our spirit. Our spirit is that which makes us alive. It is the dramatic momentum that drives our life. The story of our life is the story of our spirit. Spirit is life, life is spirit. As long as our story lives, we live.

Thumotics Clarified

Thumotics is about clearly defining the word "spirit," advocating for a general consensus on the definition, learning more about it by way of scientific study, caring for it, healing it, and developing theories and practices related to it.

Why Start with Thumos?

There are six benefits to initiating Thumotics by defining spirit in terms of Homeric *thumos*:

First, it gives a clear definition of spirit and thereby addresses the problem of not having one. Based on this clear definition, we can also have clear definitions of related words like "spiritual" and "spirituality." "Spiritual" means "of, about, related to spirit" with "spirit" clearly defined in terms of *thumos*. So, for example, "spiritual belief" refers to a belief that is of, about, or related to spirit. A "spiritual practice" is a practice that is related to our spirit. The phrase "spiritual person" would become extinct because every person, being alive, is a person of, about, or related to spirit. We cannot be a person without spirit.

"Spirituality" means "the condition of having spirit." Again, here "spirit" is defined in terms of Homeric *thumos*. Since spirit and life have a narrative quality, a spirituality is a narrative of one's spirit and life. With this clear definition we see that there is no such thing as "spirituality." Instead there are many different spiritualities. Every individual living thing has its own spirituality. Thumotic spirituality, as introduced in Chapter Eight, is the only spirituality in which spirit is clearly defined in terms of Homeric *thumos*.

Secondly, by defining spirit in terms of Homeric *thumos,* Thumotics is Western-rooted; that is, it has its roots in the cultural bedrock of Western civilization: Ancient Greece. We Westerners have no need to turn to Asian religions to fill the void of the failing, contentious, domineering Middle Eastern monotheisms (Judaism, Christianity, and Islam) that subverted and took over the West. We have deep, living roots in Ancient Greece, Rome, and Northern Europe that still nourish us. Inherent in Western civilization is an openness to ideas and practices from other cultures evaluated from our own Western perspective.

The third benefit of founding Thumotics on Homeric *thumos* is that *thumos* is nature-based rather than supernaturally or metaphysically based. It makes it possible to develop our knowledge of and practices related to spirit based on natural science rather than religious or metaphysical belief. It takes us beyond the discredited scientific theory of vitalism. Thumotics is no more vitalistic than either biology or psychology. It is a different perspective of life and a richer view of being alive in comparison to mind-body theories.

Fourthly, Thumotics is spirit-focused. It ends the reduction of life to a chemical process and the conflation of spirit with mind. Thumotics, unlike biology, is not restricted by materialism and to defining life in purely materialistic terms. Neither does it conflate spirit with mind or restrict spirit to being an aspect of mind. In Thumotics, spirit exists on its own terms. It is ontologically prior to both mind and body. A body with no spirit is a cadaver. Contrary to Descartes's "I think, therefore I am," Thumotics asserts, "Because I am alive, I think."

Fifthly, in Thumotics, since spirit is quasi-physical, it is experientially-known. It is not known by faith; that is, it is not known by believing it exists because someone in authority says it does or appeals to special, divine revelation. We can and do experience it directly. We can describe and clearly define it. As we did with the words "body" and "mind" and so many other words, we can reach a general consensus about what the word "spirit" does and does not refer to. We can have a public discussion about spirit that is more than a sharing of equally valued private opinions and beliefs. We can learn more about spirit, what it is, how to care for it in all living things, how to heal it, and how to live better lives based on our ongoing development of our knowledge of spirit.

The sixth and last benefit of basing Thumotics on Homeric *thumos*, is that in being nature-based, experientially-known, and spirit-focused, it is inherently life-affirming. It inherently affirms the value of life here, in this world, in all of nature, by acknowledging the mere fact that we are alive rather than not, by being wondered by this mere fact, by wondering more about it, by paying close attention to it, caring for it, healing it, and developing our human theories and practices related to it. In doing so, it also affirms everything that affirms life, including death. Life requires death. Death requires life. One does not exist without the other.

The next chapter spins out interesting linguistic implications of re-visioning spirit in terms of *thumos*.

4 SPIRITUAL LANGUAGE

*If you change the way you look at things,
the things you look at change.* -Wayne Dyer

Re-visioning spirit in terms of Homeric *thumos* leads to a broad re-visioning of our spirit-related language. Consider the following words related to spirit:

Spirited

Currently, spirited usually refers to being more energetic than normal. For example, a spirited horse is a horse that is more energized in comparison to its usual state and that of other horses.

Spirited also refers to being suddenly taken away. For example: In the rush of the mob, they were spirited away and vanished.

Re-visioning spirited in terms of *thumos* gives a new perspective on the word. From a Thumotic perspective, spirited simply means "has spirit." Whatever is spirited has that which makes it alive, spirit.

But being spirited also means more than being alive. Consider the difference between the following:

That oak tree is alive.

That oak tree is spirited.

The first sentence says only that the oak tree is alive rather than dead. The second sentence says that it is spirited. It has that which makes it a living rather than a dead tree. It further implies that having spirit carries with it qualities beyond the mere fact of being alive. Its qualities might include strength and fertility. When the oak tree is no longer spirited, it is also no longer strong and fertile because strength and fertility were qualities of its spirit.

Spiritual

"Spiritual" is a frequently used word. One of the fastest growing non-religious designations is "spiritual but not religious." Many have developed an allergy to the word "religious." They use "spiritual" instead.

"Spiritual" often qualifies other words as in the following sentences:

She is a very spiritual person.

His spiritual beliefs include reincarnation, past lives, and ascended masters.

Their main spiritual practice is praying for world peace.

It was a very spiritual experience.

Sedona, Arizona is one of the most spiritual places on earth.

They offer a course in spiritual guidance.

Spiritual knowledge is higher than scientific knowledge.

The book "Spiritual Growth" is on the table next to the couch.

The problem with the sentences above is that we have no general consensus on what they mean. Chances are high that, if they mean anything, they mean very different things to different people.

What is the difference, if any, between spiritual and religious?

What does it mean to be a spiritual person? How is that different from being a religious person or just a person?

How do spiritual beliefs and practices differ from religious and other beliefs and practices?

What exactly is a spiritual experience? What makes it different from other experiences?

What is a spiritual place? How do spiritual places differ from other places?

What is spiritual guidance? Is the guidance itself spiritual or is it guidance in whatever is meant by spiritual. Is it both or something else?

Is spiritual knowledge knowledge of spiritual things? If so, what are spiritual things? Is spiritual knowledge knowledge gained by spiritual means? If so, what are spiritual means?

What exactly is spiritual growth? What grows? What is it growth in and how do we do it?

What exactly do we mean when we use the word "spiritual"? Pay attention to the word. When you say it, what do you mean? When you hear it spoken or read it, are you sure you know what the other person means?

Do some add the word for affect? Do they feel the need to add some "Woo", as in "She is a very spiritual person"? Woo!

Re-Visioning "Spiritual"

Re-visioning "spiritual" in light of *thumos* gives a new perspective. In the Thumotic perspective, "spiritual" is clearly defined as "of, about, or related to that which makes alive, spirit." From the Thumotic perspective-

The difference between "spiritual" and "religious" is clear. Whatever is spiritual is of, about, or related to spirit, that which makes alive. Whatever is religious is of, about, or related to religion. We do well to stop using "spiritual" as a euphemism for "religious." Those who are religious need not be so ashamed of it that they hide behind another word.

A "spiritual person" is a person who is of, about, or related to spirit, that which makes alive. Since we must be alive to be a person and spirit is what makes us alive, "spiritual person" is somewhat redundant. There is no such thing as an unspiritual person. We are either spiritual or dead.

However, "spiritual person" can refer to a person in whom spirit stands out. It stands out rather than their body or their mind. Some have bodies that stand out rather than their minds or spirits; for example, bodybuilders. Some have minds that stand out rather than their bodies or spirits; for example, intellectuals. Others have spirits that stand out rather than their bodies or minds. We refer to them, for example, as being "mean spirited", having a "sweet spirit", or having a "presence" that fills the room. Still others might have a combination of two or all three standing out equally. A spiritual person is one in whom spirit stands out the most.

"Spiritual beliefs" are beliefs specifically "of, about, or related to spirit, that which makes alive." They are experientially and scientifically known. They have nothing to do with religious, psychic, or metaphysical beliefs. They are not known by faith but are verifiable and reasonable to believe on the basis of current, publicly shared experience and evidence.

"Spiritual practices" are specific practices "of, about, or related to that which makes alive, spirit." They are actions that, more or less, affirm or deny life. Life-affirming practices include but are not limited to breathing fresh air; eating pure, fresh, nutritious food; drinking clean, fresh water; learning; enjoying pleasures; reproducing; healing injuries and illnesses; helping others in need; doing meaningful work; resting; and sleeping.

A "spiritual experience" is an experience that is "of, about, or related to that which makes us alive, spirit." It, to a greater or lesser degree, affirms or denies that which makes us alive. Being alive, emotions, moods, fainting, illness, injury, healing, awareness of our own spirit, awareness of the spirits of others, and other experiences of, about, or related to that which makes alive are spiritual experiences.

"Spiritual place" refers to a place where that which makes alive is the outstanding characteristic. The discussion about whether or not places are spirited is beyond the scope of this brief introduction. For now, it is enough to be aware of how different places feel. Courtrooms, capitol buildings, school buildings, college campuses, church buildings, graveyards, waterfalls, valleys, mountains, parks, military bases, battlefields, hospice in-patient buildings, assisted living buildings, nursing homes, and hospitals all have different spirits. Even different places within the categories just listed have different spirits. Each place has its own unique spirit.

"Spiritual guidance" refers to guidance of another's spirit. This is discussed in more detail in Chapter Five, *Loving Care of Spirit*.

"Spiritual knowledge" refers to knowledge that is of, about, or related to that which makes alive, spirit. It is knowledge of spirit based on experience and scientific inquiry. It is not of, about, or related to anything otherworldly, supernatural, metaphysical, psychic, or religious. Neither is it knowledge gained by supernatural, religious, psychic, or metaphysical means. It is natural, not supernatural. However, Thumotics neither denies nor affirms the truth of religious, psychic, or metaphysical beliefs. They are outside the scope of Thumotics.

"Spiritual growth" could refer to growth that is of, about, or related to spirit, except that whether or not that which makes alive grows is yet to be determined. At this point, it appears that spirit, unlike body and mind, does not grow. We see that it is either present or not. We also see that we can be more or less spirited at different times; that is, spirit can vary in degree. We also see that spirit can vary in quality- mean, sweet, loving, great, strong, weak, etc.

However, we do not observe it growing and declining like our bodies. Nor do we observe it developing like our minds. Rather than growing, spirit as that which makes alive, is the agent of physical and mental growth. No spirit, no physical or mental growth.

For now, from the perspective of Thumotics, "spiritual growth" might best refer to the natural process of developing healthy instincts that help us remain alive. As we live, we learn what affirms and denies, what helps, protects, hinders, threatens, and takes our spirit, that which makes alive. Spiritual growth is the process of learning how best to stay alive and live well.

Spirituality

The word "spirituality" is in the top ten percent of popular words. Culturally, we have several serious problems regarding spirituality. The most serious is that we have no general consensus on what the word means. It can mean whatever one wants it to mean. Since we have no general consensus on what the word means, we have no coherent public conversation about it and no publicly shared knowledge of it.

Chapter Eight explores this problem in more detail and offers a Thumotic perspective.

Re-Visioning Other Words Related to Spirit

The following is a list of several other words that have spirit as their root word. They are re-visioned in the light of defining spirit in terms of Homeric *thumos*.

Aspire, to spirit toward. When we aspire to something our spirit rather than our body or mind drives us there.

Conspire, to spirit together. Those who conspire to do something, join their spirits together to do it.

Dispirit, to not-spirit, to take away spirit, deny spirit. To dispirit another is to deny and diminish their life and what makes them alive. To be dispirited is to suffer having one's spirit and life diminished and denied.

Expire, to spirit out. When spirit exits a living thing, it dies.

Inspire, to spirit in. When we inspire another, we increase their spiritedness.

Respirate, to spirit again. Respiration occurs when spirit returns after it left. Fainting and resuscitation are examples of being respirated.

Transpire, to spirit through. The story of a life, or any part of it, is the story of what transpired. What transpired is the story of what the spirited one lived through and how. The story of an entire life, of what transpired, is not just a story. It is the story of a spirit.

Re-Visioning Other Ideas

Spirit and anthropology: Anthropology has to do with the study of human beings. By re-visioning spirit Thumotics revisions what it means to be human. Essential to being human is to be spirited and alive. Being spirited has to do with the ur-drive of being human, the fundamental drive to remain spirited and alive. This drive is the drive to nourish, protect, and reproduce ourselves and others. It is fundamental to anthropology.

Spirit and body: spirit is what makes a body alive; an unspirited body is a cadaver.

Spirit and mind: spirit is what makes mind alive, spirit exists without mind in plants and non-human animals, but the human mind cannot live without spirit. Spirit precedes the mind. Before our mind develops, it is spirited. Consciousness requires spirit. No spirit, no consciousness. However, we can be spirited and unconscious, for example, in a coma.

"Meaning-making" is an act of our mind that being spirited makes possible. It is a psychological rather than a spiritual process. It is the process of cognitively identifying what is meaningful to us. Acting according to what is meaningful is optional.

Spirit and emotions: spirit is the seat of emotions. Emotions are our spirit's responses to either our actual in-the-world experiences or our thoughts and mental images. Chapter Six introduces a thumotic theory of emotions.

Spirit and moods: Moods are extended, prolonged emotions that are manifestations of our spirit. Like emotions, some moods are responses to our in-the-world experiences. Others are mind-based responses to our thoughts and mental images.

Spirit and society: A society is a unified collection of living beings. Each society has its own unique, collective spirit. Thumotics raises the question of who all is in a society. Are only human beings members of societies? Might not plants, other animals, and all living things be in a society together?

Spirit and culture: A society's culture manifests its unique, collective spirit in its language, arts, sciences, healthcare, religions, politics, laws, economic, and other aspects of culture.

Spirit and science: Science is one aspect of culture. It is an expression of a culture's spirit; specifically, its publicly shared knowledge gained by scientific research.

Spirit and art: Art is a manifestation of both an individual's and culture's spirit. It also influences the spirits of the individuals in the culture.

Spirit and politics: Politics has to do with how members of a society govern themselves and keep its members inside the defined boundaries of the society. A society's politics both manifest and shape a culture's collective spirit and the individuals of it.

Spirit and economics: Economics have to do with the goods and services produced by the members of a society. The goods and services both express and shape the individual spirits in the economy as well as the society's collective spirit and life. A society's economics shape the collective and individual spirits by either affirming or denying their life.

Spirit and medicine: Medicine is the science, art, and practice of healing. It is another manifestation of a culture's collective spirit and shaper of the spirits of its members.

Medicine that focuses on the body to the exclusion of the spirit and mind, is malpractice. It violates the fundamental rule of medicine: First, do no harm. Medicine that ignores spirit and mind does harm.

Re-visioning medicine in light of Thumotics furthers the discussions of wholistic and holistic medicine. It redefines and intensifies the importance of wholistic medicine as care of body, mind, and spirit. It further redefines and intensifies the importance of holistic medicine.

In holistic medicine, the whole is greater than the sum of its parts. A human being is greater than the sum of his or her parts. A human being is also a part of greater human wholes like family, community, business, county, state, nation, global community. Furthermore, humans are parts of other living wholes that include other animals, plants, and all living things.

The whole is affected by the parts. The parts are affected by the whole. Everything is interconnected and a whole. Everything is one by the mere fact that everything exists. From the perspective of Thumotics, the health and well-being of every living thing is profoundly related to the health and well-being of every other living thing.

The *Thumotic Lexicon* at the end of this book presents a more complete listing of words coined and re-visioned in the light of Homeric *thumos*.

The purpose of the next chapter is to inspire your love of spirit and life and wondering about how best to for your own spirit and the spirits of others.

5 LOVING CARE OF SPIRIT

I love life because what else is there? -Anthony Hopkins

Wonder of wonders! We are alive! No one told us to be alive. We didn't chose to be alive. We just are.

We are alive and we are not alone.

We are alive together. All living beings are alive together and depend on each other.

When we are healthy, we love being alive and living. Every day we naturally express our love of life by taking action to stay alive. We breathe, eat, drink, work, and rest to live. We naturally avoid pain and seek pleasure. We naturally protect ourselves from illness and injury. When ill or injured we retreat and recover. If we don't love and take care of our life, we die.

Your life matters. It matters to you if no one else. It is *your* life. If your life does not matter to you, something is wrong.

The lives of others matter too. They matter to them. They matter to you too, especially family and friends. We help each other live. If we do not, something is wrong.

The lives we take to feed our own matter. They certainly matter to those we kill for food. They also matter to us because our lives depend on them.

All our lives matter. How we live individually and collectively are life and death matters.

Spirit is life. Loving life and living are inherent to spirit. It is what spirit does. Since loving life and living are inherent to spirit, spirit inherently loves and cares for itself. Spiritual care, loving care of that which makes alive, is inherent to every living thing. Every living thing naturally cares for its own spirit and the spirit in others, unless there is something seriously wrong.

But spiritual care as "loving care of that which makes alive" is not the current view and practice of spiritual care.

The Current Reality of Spiritual Care

The current view and practice of spiritual care is this: It is caring about another human being's religious and existential concerns. It can be provided by anyone. No special training, certification, or licensure is required. However, in most government, healthcare, and other organizations Christian clergy usually provide it.

The current practice of spiritual care often includes being present, listening, referencing sacred writings, praying, and other religious practices. For those trained in existential counseling, it includes validating and normalizing questions about the meaning of life, suffering, and death as well as supporting another in his or her own "meaning-making."

Research on spiritual care in healthcare settings supports the belief that the current practice of spiritual care, regardless of which clinical discipline provides it, adds to the quality of life of patients who want to receive it and do. Those who receive support for their religious faith and practice and/or existential issues report being comforted, more accepting of their condition, and suffering less.

Since evidence supports the belief that the current practice of spiritual care relieves suffering and improves the quality of human life, we do well to continue and improve it.

However, it is misnamed. It could be improved by calling it what it is rather than half-cloaking it under words thought to make it more marketable. It is not spiritual care. It is not care of spirit. It is religious and existential care. It is care of another's religious faith, whether their religion is a traditional corporate religion or a personally created, eclectic religion. It is also care of another's existential issues, their "meaning-making." "Chaplaincy" is the best name for religious/existential care. "Chaplain" is the best name for the professionals who provide this care. Other titles such as "Spiritual Caregiver" and "Spiritual Counselor" are obvious, half-cloaked attempts to avoid an overt connection with Christianity and organized religion.

Chaplaincy could be further improved by having only licensed, board-certified chaplains provide care. Board-certified chaplains have to meet professional standards in education, training, authorization, endorsement, ethics, and continuing education. State licensure would validate their credibility to the State and taxpayers.

Additional improvement would include having chaplains care for members of their own religion. Board-certified chaplains are educated and trained in their own religion and authorized and endorsed by officials of their own religion. In a very real sense, there are no chaplains. There are Catholic chaplains, Baptist chaplains, Jewish chaplains, Muslim chaplains, Unitarian Universalist chaplains, Buddhist chaplains, New Age chaplains, Wiccan, and other chaplains. They are best qualified to care for those of their own religion.

The current practice of chaplains providing generic religious care to believers of any religion lacks integrity. It often has chaplains pretending to be something they are not: generic representatives of religion as a whole. It also often puts chaplains in conflict with their own religion by having them support religious beliefs and practices contrary to their own. More importantly, it has chaplains providing substandard care to those of faiths different from their own. Chaplains caring for those in the same religion as their own and referring those of different religions to the officials of those religions is a better practice.

Additional integrity would be gained in using the title Chaplain only for Christian clergy serving in special settings like hospice organizations, hospitals, businesses, and the military. Furthermore, the chaplain's Christian denomination needs to specified: Catholic, Baptist, Methodist, Episcopalian, Lutheran, etc. Officials of other religions have their own titles and need not be given the Christian title of Chaplain.

Finally, chaplaincy could be further improved by requiring chaplains to be licensed by the state to provide existential or any other kind of counseling outside the scope of their religion.

Re-Visioning Spiritual Care

So, if what is currently called spiritual care is not care of spirit but chaplaincy and/or existential care, what might care of spirit be?

In Thumotics, spiritual care is re-visioned, named, and clearly defined in the light of Homeric *thumos*.

The thumotic word for spiritual care is philothumy. It combines *phileo* and *thumos*. *Phileo* is an Ancient Greek word for love. *Thumos* is the Homeric word for spirit and spiritedness.

Philothumy is love of spirit, love of that which makes alive, love of life, love of being alive and living. It is loving one's own spirit and the spirits of others. It is about holding life dear and saying "Yes!" to life.

Being kind to and caring for one's own spirit and the spirits of others expresses philothumy. Helping ourselves and others live well and become what we are meant to become expresses philothumy.

Philothumy is spiritual care. It is loving care of spirit, our own and other's. It is inter- and intra-species. We care for the spirits of both our own species and those of other species too.

Philothumy is natural and inherent to being alive. Our spirit propels us to love and care for ourselves and others so that we keep living. The spirits of others propel them to care for their own and other's spirits for the same purpose. Spiritual care is our norm, something we all instinctively do. We all get better at it by adapting to our circumstances and learning from our experiences. If we do not, we die.

Spiritual care, loving care of our own spirit and life and of others is not something we *should* do. It is not an objective moral or religious law we must be ordered to obey as in "Thou shalt love the Lord thy God with all thine heart, and with all thy soul, and with all thy might" and "Love thy neighbor as thyself." It does not require command and coercion by threat of punishment.

Spiritual care is something all the living naturally do. We humans do well to recognize it, be wondered by it, affirm, support, and celebrate it. We do well to wonder about it, ask questions about it, and develop our knowledge of and skill in doing it. After all, we humans are among the youngest, if not the youngest, species of animals on Earth. We still have much to learn from others about how best to live.

Philothumy is certainly not about needlessly taking the lives of others. That is misothumy, hatred of spirit and life. Misothumy is about murder and genocide. However, since our lives require us to kill and eat other living things, we do kill and eat others in order to live. We do well to kill and eat others as respectfully and kindly as possible. We do well to feel and express deep gratitude for those who give their lives for us that we might continue to live.

Philothumy is not about self-denial or suicide so that others might live. It is not about valuing and affirming the spirit and life of others while devaluing or denying our own. It is about valuing and affirming both our own spirit and life and other's too. It is about being in mutually beneficial relationships.

At times, philothumy might involve self-denial and even suicide. But only in exceptional and extreme cases are self-denial and suicide the standards of excellence for spiritual care of others.

Philothumy is also not about doing to others as we would have them do to us. Doing to others what we want done to us is not love. It helps no one. It neither meets our own needs or the needs of others. It assumes that others want done to them what we want done to us and ignores that what others want might differ from what we want.

Rather philothumy is about taking good care of ourselves with the help of others when we need it. It is also about helping others when they cannot meet their needs on their own.

Differences Between Chaplaincy and Spiritual Care as Philothumy

There are clear differences between chaplaincy and spiritual care as philothumy.

The first difference is that chaplaincy is limited to human beings. Spiritual care is not. As far as we now know, only humans have religions and need religious officials to help them with their religious concerns. Only humans have existential concerns and need help with them. Spiritual care, loving care of spirit, applies to all living things. All healthy living things naturally love and care for their own spirit and the spirits of others.

The second difference between chaplaincy and spiritual care is what is cared for. Chaplaincy focuses on religious and existential concerns. Spiritual care focuses on spirit, that which makes alive. It is possible to focus on a person's religious beliefs and practices without regard for the person's spirit or life. Caring for another's spirit, requires regard for the whole living being and its whole life.

The third difference is that religious professionals, chaplains, provide chaplaincy. All healthy living things love and care for spirit, their own and other's. Spiritual care as philothumy is inherent and natural to all living things.

The fourth difference between chaplaincy and spiritual care as philothumy has to do with spiritual guidance.

From Spiritual Care to Spiritual Guidance: Thumogogy

Currently, spiritual guidance is a specialty within the broader scope of religious care. Spiritual guidance, like religious care, is often provided by religious officials or laity with special training. It focuses on guiding clients in their religious faith and practice.

Spiritual guidance requires knowledge of religious teachings and practices and, in its modern liberal forms, psychology and counseling. The skills of spiritual guidance include being present, listening, asking open-ended questions, validating and normalizing experiences, teaching, reflecting on thoughts, feelings, and actions, citing sacred writings, encouraging, giving specific directions to follow, praying, and other religious practices.
It focuses not on guiding a person's spirit. It focuses on individuals' religious experiences and becoming more faithful in the beliefs and practices of their religion.

In Thumotics, spiritual guidance is re-visioned in the light of philothumy. It is named thumogogy. Thumogogy combines *thumos* and *agogos,* meaning leader or guide. It refers to spiritual guidance in the sense of guiding and leading another's spirit from one mode of being to another.

While philothumy is loving, befriending, and caring for one's own spirit and the spirits of others, thumogogy is a more active and intentional guidance of another's spirit in the process of fulfilling its life-affirming desires.

Thumogogy expresses the values and practices of being wondered by and wondering about life, humility, holistic knowing, and harmony.

Thumogogy requires knowledge of spirit (thumology), thumic norms, spiritual health and illness, the various conditions of spirit, emotions of spirit, how to connect spirit to spirit, and what affects and changes spirit.

The skills of thumogogy include the skills of being present, listening, asking open-ended questions, validating and normalizing experiences, connecting with the other's spirit, teaching about spirit, coaching and reflecting on thoughts, feelings and actions, encouraging, and, most important of all, setting an example.

The goal of thumogogy is to guide another's spirit from where it is to a healthier condition.

The process begins with creating a safe space for the client, connecting with the client spirit to spirit, feeling and discerning the client's spirit, and assessing the current reality of the client's spirit.

It continues with identifying the life-affirming desires of the client's heart, how the client is doing with fulfilling them, creating a plan of care together, implementing the plan, continuing or revising the plan of care until the client's goal is reached.

The process of spiritual guidance ends when the client reaches his or her goal.

Our loving care of our own spirit and the spirits of others inspires us to know more and better understand spirit. The next chapter presents a brief introduction to spiritual knowledge re-visioned.

6 SPIRITUAL KNOWLEDGE

Basically, I have been compelled by curiosity. -Mary Leaky

Because we naturally love life and that which makes us alive, spirit, we also naturally love learning more about life and that which makes us alive.

Loving life, being wondered by the mere fact of being alive rather than not, inspires our natural curiosity and wondering about spirit. Curiosity is inherent to spirit. It is our urge to draw near and discover more.

It rises up in our mind as questions that ache for answers: Why are we alive rather than not? What does it mean to be alive? What makes us alive rather than not?

Living with these and other related questions, gathering and remembering experiences and information, and forming tentative answers, gives us knowledge. However, we are human. Our knowledge is limited and tentative. It is always open to revision due to new discoveries and learning.

This chapter is about our spiritual knowledge. It reviews current perspectives of spiritual knowledge. It also introduces thumology, a re-visioning of spiritual knowledge in terms of Homeric *thumos*.

Current Perspectives of Spiritual Knowledge

As with the words "spirit" and "spiritual", we have no general consensus on a clear definition of "spiritual knowledge." "Spiritual knowledge" can refer to rational knowledge of religious doctrine, experiential knowledge of supernatural/metaphysical realms and beings, knowledge and practice of religious/metaphysical practices like prayer, devotional reading, chanting, meditation, fasting, following dietary guidelines, abstaining from sex, not bearing children, abstaining from physical pleasures, and practicing poverty and dependence on others. "Spiritual knowledge" can also refer to knowledge gained by psychic or occult means such as clairvoyance or divination.

Examples of people referred to as having spiritual knowledge include the Pope, the Dali Lama, priests, pastors, rabbis, imams, mystics, monks, nuns, shamans, psychics, mediums, astrologers, and New Age celebrities. Generally speaking, "spiritual knowledge" is currently knowledge that we cannot verify for ourselves but must accept by faith.

To be clear, from the perspective of Thumotics, there is no denial of the veracity of the claims to "spiritual knowledge" as described above. Such claims are outside the scope of and irrelevant to Thumotics.

Spiritual Knowledge Re-Visioned

With the re-visioning of "spirit" as "that which makes alive" and "spiritual" as "of, about, or related to spirit", we can have a shared, public conversation in which we talk about the same things when we use these words.

On the basis of a general consensus about the meaning of "spiritual", we can revision what we mean by "spiritual knowledge. "Spiritual knowledge" now refers to " knowledge of, about, or related to spirit, that which makes alive." Now we can base our knowledge of spirit on the scientific study of spirit.

The thumotic word for the scientific study of spirit is thumology. It is based on *thumos* and *logos* and means "the study of *thumos*." As *bios* is to biology and *psyche* is to psychology, so *thumos* is to thumology.

Thumology

Since spirit re-visioned in the light of Homeric *thumos* is quasi-physical and in the natural rather than supernatural realm, we can base our knowledge of spirit on scientific study. Thumology, the scientific study of spirit, is professional and amateur wondering about spirit. It is an act of natural curiosity and philothumy. It begins with being wondered by the fact of being alive rather than not. It continues with wondering about being alive rather than not.

As biologists study physical life and psychologists study the human psyche or mind, thumologists study spirit.

The questions thumologists explore include but are not limited to the following: Why study spirit? What is spirit? What are its characteristics? What is its anatomy? What is a healthy spirit? What is an ill or injured spirit? What are its conditions? What harms and what heals the spirit?

Why Study Spirit?

Studying spirit is an act of love. It is our spirit's natural response to our love of life and being wondered by the mere fact of being alive rather than not. The mere fact of being alive inspires our spirit's curiosity to know more about being alive. Our curiosity inspires questions in our mind and urges us to seek answers. As we engage in the curious process of gathering information, asking questions, and forming answers we gain knowledge. Our knowledge is an ongoing, organic, ever-changing process based on our perspective at the time.

Studying spirit is also a natural drive of our spirit because remaining alive is an inherent drive of spirit. It compels our mind to learn more about spirit so that we may overcome threats to our spirit and life and keep living.

Current Reality of the Scientific Study of Spirit

Currently, Western science does not study spirit understood in terms of *thumos*. It functions within the parameters of materialism, rationalism, and dualism. Since Western science assumes that spirit is a religious/metaphysical/supernatural concept that one can believe in or not, it either dismisses spirit as being outside its scope or simply denies its existence altogether.

Where We Need to Go

We Westerners suffer greatly due to our lack of scientific study of spirit. Re-visioning spirit in the light of Homeric *thumos* includes it in the realm of nature and, therefore, within the scope of the natural sciences.

We need scientists devoted to the study of spirit defined in terms of Homeric *thumos*. We need them now. Our spirit- and life-denying ways are wreaking havoc on our own lives, the lives of countless others, and entire species. How we are living now is unsustainable.

We need to know more about spirit. We need to better understand it so that we can make better decisions on how to take good care of our own individual spirits, the spirits of others, and spirits of groups.

How We Get There: Thumologists and Thumonauts

Thumologists will be the ones who establish and develop the scientific study of spirit. We need some who are well-trained in scientific study to step forward, be the first thumologists, lay the foundation of thumology, and lead the way in its development. Our need is urgent. It will take generations for thumology to have a meaningful impact on Western society and the world. We need its impact sooner rather than later.

We need thumologists to prove their work quickly and initiate interdisciplinary study with physicists, biologists, anthropologists, historians, philologists, psychologists, thanatologists, and others.

We need them engaged in holistic knowing that affirms empirical, deductive, intuitive, gut-brain, anecdotal, and thumotic knowing.

To gather information for thumologists to analyze and understand, we also need thumonauts, trained observers and explorers of spirit. We need thumonauts exploring the uncharted realms of the human spirit, gathering data, and feeding it to thumologists to analyze, form theories, and do further research.

What is Spirit?

The fundamental question of thumology is this: What is spirit?

The Thumotic perspective introduced here defines spirit in terms of Homeric *thumos*. In its simplest terms, it defines spirit as "that which makes alive." It proposes this definition as a place to start, not the final authoritative answer. As we practice thumonautics and thumology, and learn more about spirit, we will articulate new iterations of its definition.

Answers to Questions About Being Alive

Over the centuries, we Westerners have developed four basic different answers to the questions of what makes something alive rather than not: materialism, hylomorphism, vitalism, and metaphysicalism.

Materialism

Materialism is a type of monism first developed in Ancient Greece by Leucippus (5th century BCE) and Democritus (died c. 370 BCE) that influences how modern Western scientists and we Westerners in general view existence and life today. It is the belief that everything consists of particles of matter, atoms. In its modern form, everything consists of waves and/or particles of energy.

Consider scientists. Some scientists believe there is more to reality than matter. Some are agnostic concerning the existence of anything other than matter. Others believe that everything that exists is matter. Regardless of their personal beliefs, in their work scientists generally function as atheistic, monistic materialists. They use the scientific method to study physical matter as if only physical matter exists.

Biologists, the scientists who study living physical things, divide physical things into two basic categories: living and non-living. From their scientific perspective living things have certain characteristics that non-living things do not. Biologists do not have one list of characteristics that they all agree on, but the following is a representative list. According to biologists, all living things have seven characteristics. They-

1. Are cells

2. Metabolize, use energy
3. Maintain internal homeostasis
4. Grow
5. Respond to stimulation
6. Adapt to their environment
7. Reproduce

Note that these are *physical* characteristics of living physical things. They are observable *characteristics*. Note also that, except for the first, all of the physical characteristics are physical *functions*.

What does it mean to be alive? What is the difference between being alive and not? Biologists give a functional answer. Living things physically function in seven or more ways that differ from non-living things.

The list of physical functions and characteristics also defines the *scope* of what biologists study. Their scope is limited by their presupposition of materialism: what exists is matter alone.

What makes us alive rather than not? Since biologists restrict their study to physical things, they answer within the scope of materialism. Their answer: a chemical process. "Chemical process" is another name for one of the characteristics of living things: metabolism. It is like saying that what makes something alive is having the characteristic of being alive. It does not answer the question of *what* makes something alive. In order to have the characteristic and function of metabolism, we must first be alive. Being alive is ontologically prior to metabolizing.

Honest biologists admit that they do not yet know *what* makes something alive rather than not. Their study continues. They also admit that they do not yet know *how* life started, *when*, or how *long* it might continue.

Hylomorphism

Hylomorphism is a type of materialistic philosophical theory developed by Aristotle (died 322 BCE), which conceives being as a compound of matter and form. Matter is what things are made of. Form is their structure. For example, a table's matter is wood. Its form is that of table: a top with legs. Both the table's matter and form are inherent to it being a table.

According to this theory, we human beings consist of body and soul. Body (*soma*) is our matter; soul (*psyche*) is our form.

What does it mean to be alive? What is the difference between being alive and not? What makes us alive? Hylomorphists believe that to be alive is to be a compound of body and soul. The difference between being alive and not is being a compound of body and soul or not.

Aristotle further believed that there are different kinds of souls: plant, animal, and human. The human soul has *nous*, intellect. Plant and animal souls do not. A human body without human soul is neither alive nor human. There is no such thing as a human soul without a body. To be a human being we must be a compound of human body and human soul. Likewise, for plant and animals.

Vitalism

Vitalism is a derogatory term used by monistic materialists for a type of dualistic scientific hypothesis that posits the metaphysical theory that physical living organisms are fundamentally different from non-living entities because they are made alive by a separate, non-physical, vitalizing energy, often called soul.

Proponents of vitalism are influenced by the dualistic philosophy of Rene Descartes (died in 1650 BCE). They believe that what makes us alive is a non-physical, life-giving force that exists apart from the physical body. This vital force is given different names like élan vital, vital spark, energy, odic force, mind, and soul.

Vitalism is alive and well among many complementary and alternative medicine practitioners who do "energy work" and work to address problems in the "bio-energy field."

Metaphysicalism

Metaphysicalism is the belief, either monistic or dualistic, that the non-physical is ontologically and axiologically prior to the physical and what makes us alive. In its monistic form, everything is "spirit" or "energy" in different degrees of thickness. In its dualistic form, everything physical comes from a non-physical source that is prior to and above the physical. This source is called by many names: God, Goddess, Creator, Spirit, Brahma, the field of pure potentially, Universe, or Source to list some of the more popular names.

Consider religious believers. Generally speaking, Western monotheists- Jews, Christians, Muslims, and others- share the dualistic belief in physical and "spiritual" (invisible, non-physical, beyond the physical) worlds. They share the belief with biologists that some things are alive and some are not. However, they believe that some living things are non-physical; for example, human souls after death, angels, and demons.

They believe a non-physical, divine being created or is the source of all things living and non-living, visible and invisible.

What does it mean to be alive? For religious believers, it means we come from a divine source. What makes us alive rather than not? The act of a divine being. What is the difference between being alive and not? The act of a divine being.

A Different Answer

What does it mean to be alive? What is the difference between being alive and not?

Thumology proposes a different answer: what makes something alive is spirit. The difference between being alive or not is spirit.

Spirit is natural, not supernatural or divine. It is quasi-physical, not metaphysical. In humans, spirit is located between the breasts and behind the breast bone. It not only makes us alive rather than not, it is our drive to live. It compels us to provide for and protect our own life and the lives of others. We can physically feel it in ourselves and others. Our emotions, moods, and characteristics are of our spirit. We can also deliberate with and influence our spirit. It can be healthy, ill, wounded, or broken. When it is broken, death often occurs.

Spirit makes everything that is alive alive. Things that are alive are dynamic, organic, chronologically changing wholes. In thumology, living, dynamic, changing wholes are called thumotic holons.

Thumotic holons are experientially perceivable wholes that change over time at relatively different rates of speed. For example, everything that biologists identify as being alive, from the smallest to the largest and simplest to most complex, is a thumotic holon. However, the concept of thumotic holons is far more inclusive. For example, it includes geological formations like rocks, mountains, and valleys that change at relatively slow rates of speed; bodies of water like springs, rivers, lakes, and oceans. Winds, fires, plants, animals (including human beings), events like dramas, parades, musical performances, and rituals, creations like buildings, statues, paintings, photographs, jewelry, and clothing are all thumotic holons.

"Spirit" refers to the dynamic, organic, chronologically changing feature of thumotic holons. We know that it exists because we experience ourselves and others being spirited. We are alive and spirit is that which makes us alive. What is the difference between a living or dead tree, honey bee, crow, wolf, cat, horse, or human being? The difference between being alive or dead is spirit.

From the perspective of thumology, as long as a thumotic holon remains an identifiable holon, it is spirited and alive. Death is not the end of a thumotic holon, rather it is the chronological moment that the holon shifts from being internally spirited (endothumotic) to being externally spirited (exothumotic).

For example, a thumotic holon that is a tree is alive when it is endothumotic. It is spirited from within. After it dies, a dead tree remains a holon because it remains identifiable as a tree. It remains spirited because it still has a dynamic, organic, chronologically changing feature. It is decaying. However, this feature does not come from within the tree but from without. It is exothumotic, externally-spirited. It remains a spirited thumotic holon until it is no longer identifiable as a tree.

The thumological perspective differs from the materialistic, hylomorphic, vitalistic, and metaphysical perspectives previously described. The materialistic perspective has two distinct categories: living and non-living. In the thumological perspective, everything that exists as a thumotic holon is spirited and alive, either endothumotically or exothumotically.

The hylomorphic perspective posits different souls for plants, non-human animals, and humans. It also asserts that a human being, for example, is no longer human after it dies. In the thumological perspective, there are not different kinds of spirits making plants, non-human animals, and humans alive. Whatever is alive is made alive by spirit. Furthermore, even after a living being dies, it remains as long as it is the identifiable holon that it has been. Contrary to hylomorphism, a dead human being is still a human being.

The vitalistic perspective posits a non-physical life-giving thing that gives life to physical things. It is a dualistic perspective that sees existence in physical and non-physical terms. The thumological perspective is monistic. It sees existence as a whole. Nature is everything that exists. That which makes alive, spirit, is as much a part of the natural, physical world as rocks, rivers, and red-heads. If divine beings exist, they are thumotic holons, part of nature, and outside the scope of what we can perceive with our physical senses.

How We Know Spirit

Another fundamental question of thumology is this: How do we know spirit? What follows is a tentative answer. It is a place to start.

We know spirit by way of induction based on our physical senses. Since it is quasi-physical, we can feel our own spirit. We can also develop tools that will record it in others.

We know it by way of deduction based on our mind's logic and mental images. In order to develop our spiritual knowledge deductively, we will have to move past the monocrats of our minds that either dismiss the existence of spirit or refuse to think of it in terms other than religious or metaphysical.

We know spirit by way of our social communications with others, the accumulation of anecdotal evidence. For example, we are aware of experiences of esprit de corps, familial spirits (the spirit of a child being similar to or the same as a parent's or grandparent's), kindred spirits (spirits of those not biologically related being similar or the same), spiritual community in which kindred spirits unite around a common interest, and spiritual communion in which two or more experience sharing the same spirit. The frequency of these experiences warrants further study.

We also know spirit by our spirit. We refer to our spirit's knowing as empathy, intuition, and direct perception. It is based on spirit-to-spirit connections. Examples of direct spirit-to-spirit knowing include "feeling" another's presence apart from our physical senses. This experience is common in some forms of martial arts. Feeling another's emotions as one's own, experiencing another as being mean, loving, warm, cold, closed, opened, or great spirited, and directly feeling another to be high- or low-spirited are also examples of directly knowing spirit.

What We Know About the Human Spirit

We know we are spirited, alive.

We know we expire, spirit out, and die.

We also know that we sustain the ongoing life of our species by way of sexual intercourse, conception, gestation, birth, and nurturing to adulthood.

These are the three great wonders and mysteries of life: life, sex, and death.

We also know that we experience ourselves as being more or less spirited at different times. Our spiritedness varies.

We know that our spiritedness varies from person to person and that we have different types of spirits. Some of us have spirits that fill the room; others do not. Some of us have loving spirits; others are mean spirited. Some of us have warm spirits; others have spirits that are cold.

We also know that our spirit can be wounded, sick, or broken. We know we can die from a broken spirit.

More is said about wounded, sick, and broken spirits in Chapter Seven on spiritual healing. What follows is a partial list of different types of human spirits. The *Thumotic Lexicon* at the back of this book lists additional types. The list is only a place to start. We will revise it as we engage in the scientific study of spirit and learn more about it.

Some Types of Human Spirits

Cryothumia: cold-spiritedness. "She has ice in her veins" expresses this type of spirit.

Dethumia: negated-spiritedness. This condition is the result of one's spirit and life being denied by oneself, others, or life-denying circumstances.

Dynathumia: strong-spiritedness, powerful, able to get things done. We refer to strong-spirited individuals as "a force of nature", "a real dynamo." Rosa Parks is one example. Eleanor Roosevelt is another.

Fellarothumia: sucking-spiritedness. These are individuals who drain the life (spirit) out of others. We refer to them with these phrases: "She sucks the life right out of me." "Just being with him makes me tired."

Glycothumia: sweet-spiritedness. This type of spirit is nice, kind, and pleasant. We say of individuals with this type of spirit, "She has such a sweet spirit." "He had the sweetest spirit about him."

Malthumia: mean-spiritedness. Mean-spirited individuals say and do things that harm or kill others. They deny the spirits of others.

Megathumia: great-spiritedness. Those with great spirits have palpable presence. Their presence can "fill a room." They can have wide-spread, historical influence. Examples of great-spirited individuals include Alexander the Great, Caesar Augustus, Catherine the Great, Albert Einstein, Martin Luther King, Jr, and Maya Angelou.

Photothumia: light-spiritedness. Those with bright spirits might be nicknamed "Sunshine" or "Sunny." They brighten the room when they walk in. They have a "sunny disposition." Bet Milder is one example.

Toxothumia: toxic-spiritedness. This type leaves others feeling like they were infected by some kind of toxin. We might say they have a "high ick factor" about them of feel "icky."

Identifying Our Thumic Norm

Our thumic norm is how our spirit is most of the time. It might or might not be how we want our spirit to be. It is how it actually is most of the time.

Use the following tool to help identify your thumic norm:

My spirit is normally-

Very Low <--> Very High

1   2   3   4   5

Very Introverted <--> Very Extroverted

1   2   3   4   5

Very Troubled <---> Very Well

1   2   3   4   5

Use up to three words or phrases that best describe how your spirit is most of the time. For example, intense, caring, and strong; social, the life of party, sunny; calm, caring, wise.

1. _____

2. _____

3. _____

To what degree are your spirit and circumstances in sync?

Not at all <---> Perfect fit

1   2   3   4   5

Explanation

The Low/High scale provides a reading of the *degree* of our spiritedness. Are we normally low-spirited, high-spirited, or somewhere in between? NOTE: In this context "Low" is descriptive. It has to do with our degree of aliveness rather than our mood.

The Introverted/Extroverted scale provides a reading of the normal *orientation* of our spirit. Is our spirit directed inward to ourselves, our thinking, imagining, and/or emotional processes; outward toward people, places, things, and events; and to what degree?

The Troubled/Well scale helps us assess the normal *overall health* of our spirit. Are we normally ill-spirited, well-spirited, or somewhere in between?

The words that best describe how our spirit is most of the time, add individuality to the verbal portrait of our thumic norm.

Finally, the degree to which our spirit and circumstances are in sync gives insight into the social context of our spirit and life.

Sample Applications

Determining our thumic norm is helpful in at least three ways. First, once we determine our thumic norm, we have a baseline with which we can compare it with other possibilities and decide if we can and want to work on changing our thumic norm.

For example, we might determine that our thumic norm is high, extroverted, troubled, and out of sync with our circumstances. We can then examine the consequences that we experience with our thumic norm and decide if we want to make some changes.

Secondly, determining our thumic norm makes it possible for us to better identify conditions of our spirit that are not our norm.

For example, if our thumic norm is somewhat low, somewhat introverted, well, and in sync with our circumstances and it changes to more extroverted and troubled, we have something to pay attention to.

Thirdly, determining our thumic norm makes it possible for us to compare our norm with our circumstances and assess if our norm and our circumstances synchronize or not. When they synchronize, we are likely to live effectively in our circumstances. When they are at odds, we can determine if we can adapt or not. If we can adapt, knowing our thumic norm and what our circumstances require, gives us insight into how we need to adapt. Knowing how we need to adapt helps us determine if we are willing and able to do so.

For example, is our thumic norm is high, introverted, well, and somewhat in sync, but our job requires us to be high, extroverted, well and in sync with it, then we have some decisions to make. How long can we sustain the demand? Can we effectively set boundaries on our job and do it from our thumic norm? Do we need to change jobs?

Whatever our thumotic norm, every day we experience waves of emotions. They arise, wash over us, and pass on. What follows is a thumotic theory of emotions.

A Thumological Theory of Emotions

To understand our emotions, it can be helpful to begin with the etymology of the word.

Our word "emotion" comes from Old French *émouvoir* "stir up" which comes from Latin *emovere* "move out, remove, agitate." *Emovere* is the combination of *ex-* "out" and *movere* "to move."

The concrete image of emotion is of something being stirred up and moving outward. For example, when we stir up sediment with a stick from the bottom of a pond, the sediment spreads and moves throughout the pond.

The first recorded use of "emotion" to refer to a strong inner feeling was in the 1650s. By 1808 it referred to any inner feeling.

In other words, "emotion" originally referred to concrete, external movements and stirrings and was later applied metaphorically to the inner up stirrings we now call our emotions. Its metaphorical use is relatively recent and modern and aptly expresses how we experience our emotions.

So, what exactly is moved and stirred up when we feel emotions?

Is our mind stirred up? If our mind is stirred up, it is with thoughts and images rather than emotions. Our thoughts and mental images can be *about* our emotions. For example, we can wonder about why we feel the emotion we feel at the time. Our thoughts and mental images can also *cause* our emotions. For example, we can image something horrible happening to us in the future and think about it happening. We can then feel fear in response to our own mental images and thoughts. But our emotions do not move out from our mind.

Is our body stirred up? Our body can respond to our emotions. For example, when we feel angry our face can flush and our muscles tense. Our body can also cause emotions. When we accidentally cut our finger, we can feel alarmed and fearful. But our emotions do not move out from our body.

From the thumological perspective, our emotions are stirrings of our spirit. In response to stimulation of our own body, mind, spirit, interactions with others; our spirit is stirred, moved, or agitated and moves from within us, through our mind and body, outward to be expressed in our words and physical actions.

More precisely, our spirit, that which makes us alive, responds to stimuli that either affirm or deny it.

Stimuli that affirm our spirit, support and sustain our spirit and our life. We welcome such stimuli and call such stirrings joy, happiness, gratitude, excitement, fear, guilt, and sorrow. When we feel such stirrings we feel more alive, more spirited.

Stimuli that deny our spirit, suppress and threaten our spirit and life. We resist such stimuli and call such stirrings fear, anger, sadness, guilt, loneliness, and despair. When we feel such stirrings we feel less alive, less spirited.

Our emotions are less about our minds and psychology and more about our spirits and thumology.

Ten Basic Emotions

The thumological theory of emotions introduced here, identifies ten basic emotions of our spirit paired as follows:

Fear and contentment
Anger and guilt
Sadness and gladness
Disgust and desire
Disappointment and gratitude

Fear is our spirit's response to danger and contentment is its response to safety.

Anger is our spirit's response to being wronged and guilt is its response to doing wrong.

Sadness is our spirit's response to loss and gladness is its response to gain.

Disgust is our spirit's response to what repels it and desire is its response to what attracts it.

Disappointment is our spirit's response to desire denied and gratitude is its response to desire relieved.

Our emotions, at their best, are our spirit's life-affirming responses to our in-the-world interactions. They show us what harms and helps our spirit and life. They are our spirit protecting and promoting itself in order to keep living and fulfill its purpose.

At their worse, our emotions are disordered, life-denying responses of our spirit to our own thoughts and imaginings. Such responses inspire us to deny our own life and hinder us in fulfilling the life-affirming desires of our hearts.

One example of a disordered emotion is an addiction to a substance that endangers our spiritual, physical, mental, and social health. From a thumological perspective, substance addiction occurs when our spirit experiences the substance as life-affirming when it actually harms and denies our life. The spirit experiences the substance-induced pleasure as life-affirming and desires it, the body craves it, and the mind is powerless to stop the behavior of consuming the substance in spite of the evidence that it is poisonous.

The distinction between the spirit's emotional responses to in-the-world interactions and mind-based thoughts and imaginings is a key feature of the thumological theory of emotions.

It is beyond the scope of this brief introduction to go into more detail on the thumological theory of emotions. A future book will go into more detail about each of the ten emotions, their quasi-physical characteristics, the life-affirming functions, and the differences between the spirit's emotional responses to actual in-life-world experiences versus its emotional responses to mind-based thoughts and imaginings.

We have so much to learn about spirit that its study will require several branches of thumology.

Branches of Thumology

Just as other sciences have different branches, even now we can imagine the different branches that we need to create. For example-

Human clinical thumology studies individuals who exhibit disorders of spirit to learn more about spiritual illnesses and injuries and how best to help those who have them.

Counseling thumology studies how to help people live the best life they can.

Human developmental thumology focuses on the spirit in humans as they develop from birth to death.

Experimental thumology focuses on the effects of physical, mental, and social interactions with spirit and vice versa.

Family thumology concentrates on the spirits of families, their characteristics, and how they affect the lives of individual family members and others.

Forensic thumologists study the spirits of criminal individuals and groups.

Geriatric thumology focuses on the spiritual health and well-being of older people.

Organizational thumology studies the human spirit in the context of work.

Physiological thumology studies the relationship between the human spirit and body

Psychological thumology studies the relationship between the human mind and spirit.

Thumometrics focuses on thumological testing and assessment.

School thumology focuses on the spiritual and emotional health of young people in educational settings.

Social thumology explores the dimension of spirit in all aspects of how we live with others on this planet.

Sports thumologists concentrate on the role of spirit in professional or amateur athletes.

Thumology comes from our love of life, wonder, and natural curiosity to know more. The knowledge gained informs our loving care of spirit. It also informs our natural desire to heal ill and injured spirits. The next chapter presents a brief introduction to spiritual healing from a thumotic perspective.

7 SPIRITUAL HEALING

The most spiritual human beings, assuming they are the most courageous, also experience by far the most painful tragedies: but it is precisely for this reason that they honor life, because it brings against them its most formidable weapons.
- Friedrich Nietzsche

Being wondered by the mere fact of being alive rather than not inspires our love of life and curiosity. We love being alive, wonder about it, and want to know more. Knowing more about being alive fans the flame of our love of life even brighter.

As we learn about and love life more, we become more aware of how every living thing struggles to keep living. We all struggle to eat, drink, protect ourselves and those we care about, and enjoy pleasure. In our struggle to keep living, none avoid illness and injury.

We are wondered by the fact that some recover from their illnesses and injuries and some do not. Some die from illnesses and injuries. Some heal partially. Some completely.

Some are killed and eaten. Others kill and eat. All desire to remain alive and struggle to do so to the end. In the end, all die and become food for the living.

We might be wondered by the fragility of some and resiliency of others. Why do some heal completely, others partially, and others die? What is healing? How do those who heal completely or partially do so? What helps them heal?

Health and Healing

To be healthy is to be whole, sound, and well in spirit, body, mind and relationships. More accurately, it is wholeness of spiritbodymind in life-affirming relationships with others. It includes being safe, prosperous, and happy. Health is not a given. Some are conceived and die in their mother's womb. Some are born unhealthy and die soon after birth. Others are born unhealthy and yet live.

All the living who become adults work and struggle to remain alive. At times we become ill or injured and need to heal.

Healing is the process of becoming whole, sound, and well again. It is the process of becoming again a whole spiritbodymind in life-affirming relationships. It is the reuniting of what belongs together and the separation of what does not. It is the reuniting of a broken bone, cut skin, a divided mind, split relationships, or a broken spirit. It is the separation and removal of a limb that cannot be mended or the end of a relationship that cannot be reconciled.

Healing is a natural process. It is like breathing. We do not choose to do it. We just do it.

When we break a bone, we immediately begin the process of healing it. When we cut ourselves, we bleed, cleanse the cut, scab, and begin the process of healing. When the narrative of our life is fragmented and makes no rational sense, we naturally think about how to connect the incoherent parts so the plot of our life is no longer broken but whole. When a relationship with someone or something we love is broken, we grieve and seek to fill the void and make ourselves whole again. When our life is denied and our spirit wounded or broken, we naturally take action to make our spirit and life whole again.

Any physical, mental, social, or spiritual injury or illness is injury and illness of the whole spiritbodymind. Beyond that, it is illness and injury of all the living.

The natural process of healing is work. It is our work, the combined work of our spiritbodymind in relationships with others.

For the work of healing, we naturally withdraw from our normal activities. When physically injured, we cleanse and bind the wound. When ill, we change both what and how much we eat. Whether ill or injured, peaceful, quiet, comfortable rest usually supports our natural healing process.

Both the injury or illness and the work of healing weaken us. Healing requires patience. It takes time to recover our strength and return to our normal activities. Impatience impedes our healing. So do discouraging thoughts. Returning to our normal activities before we have sufficiently recovered only puts us and others at risk of additional harm.

The severity of the harm we suffer, along with our condition at the time of the illness or injury, determine how long it takes us to heal and return to our normal activities. We know we are nearing recovery when our spirit urges us to eat, drink, move around, think encouraging and life-affirming words, and gradually return to our normal activities.

We observe the same general, natural process of healing in all living things.

Therapy

Even though our healing is a natural process we do ourselves, sometimes we need help with our healing. Sometimes we need therapy.

"Therapy" comes from the Ancient Greek word *therapeuien*, "to attend, do service, take care of." A therapist is someone who attends to, serves, and takes care of us while we heal. Therapists do not heal us. We heal ourselves. Therapists attend to, serve, and take good care of us while we do our own work of healing.

By supporting us during our natural healing work, therapists lighten the burden of our healing work. Thereby they make it possible for us to heal quicker and more completely. As a result, we return sooner to our normal activities of living than we would without therapy.

Different kinds of therapists help us with different kinds of healing. Currently, physicians are usually our primary attendants. Sometimes they refer us to other therapists; for example, physical therapists, respiratory therapists, and psychotherapists.

We have a general consensus on what the words "Doctor," "physician," "physical therapy," "respiratory therapy," and "psychotherapy" refer to. They do not refer to whatever we privately believe. They have relatively narrow, publicly understood ranges of meaning and make it possible to have coherent conversations about them.

Spiritual Healing

But what about "spiritual healing" and "spiritual therapy"? What do these words mean? To what do they refer?

"Spiritual healing" is part of our vocabulary, but we have no general consensus on what the words mean. For some, spiritual healing is healing *of* a person's inner self or soul. It might involve the healing of one's past life, becoming enlightened, having one's soul saved from damnation, finding one's purpose, escaping the cycle of reincarnation, or ascension to a higher vibration or level of consciousness.

For some, spiritual healing is healing *by* non-medical, religious, metaphysical, or psychic means. The means of spiritual healing might be prayer, meditation, receiving healing energy, a shamanic journey, guided imagery, past life regression, connecting with one's Higher Self, crystals, or gaining insight through a form of divination.

For others, spiritual healing is healing *from* a supernatural or divine being such as a god, goddess, the Buddha, Jesus, a bodhisattva, angel, saint, or ascended master.

For still others, spiritual healing is something else.

Note that none of the above definitions of spiritual healing are clearly "of, about, or related to spirit."

Since we Westerners have no general consensus on what spiritual healing is, we suffer from the lack of it.

Spiritual Healing Re-visioned

In Thumotics, spirit is re-visioned and clearly defined in terms of Homeric *thumos*. So is spiritual healing.

Our spirit is that which makes us alive rather than not. It is that which drives us to remain alive and healthy. It is an organic, unfolding narrative.

Before we can understand spiritual healing, we need a clear definition of a healthy spirit, euthumia. Only then can we begin to identify when our spirit is ill or injured spirit and needs to heal. The following nine characteristics of euthumia serve as a working definition and place to start.

Nine Characteristics of Euthumia

A healthy spirit is-

1. Relatively well and whole, unwounded, unbroken. Neither spiritual, physical, mental, or social problems hinder one's relative quality of life. This does not mean that we never experience challenges, injury, illness, or harm. It means that such challenges do not significantly hinder the wholeness and effectiveness of our life.

2. Free to live and become what one is meant to become, able to determine one's own life, not restricted by economic, political, social, or other external limitations.

3. Self-motivated to live and continue becoming what one is meant to become.

4. Self-supporting, able to sustain the unfolding narrative of one's spirit and life, able to provide for oneself food, drink, and protection.

5. Connected harmoniously with others, able to communicate effectively with others and help sustain the lives of others.

6. Willing and able to face life's challenges rather than avoid them or seek escape.

7. Creative, productive, and able to solve the problems that challenge living, and contribute to the lives of others.

8. Successful in life's endeavors, learns from experiences, and fulfills desires.

9. Respectful of others, lives one's life and does not interfere unnecessarily with others living theirs.

These nine characteristics are not absolutes. They vary throughout the unfolding of our life. They are general characteristics of euthumia, not moral imperatives for what we should and ought to do. They are the behaviors of healthy living things. We observe these behaviors in the stories of well, uninjured living things. Those that engage in these behaviors, suffer less and live longer than those who do not.

The nine characteristics of euthumia give us a working definition and standard by which to identify and measure spiritual healthiness and unhealthiness. The thumotic word for spiritual unhealthiness is dysthumia. When we lack one or more of the nine characteristics of euthumia, we are either ill or injured. The health of our spirit needs to be restored or we die.

When we are dysthumic, we are spiritually ill or injured and our ability to keep living is challenged. When our spirit is ill or injured, so are our body and mind. When our body and mind are harmed, so is our spirit. We live as a whole spiritbodymind in relationships with everything else. What harms a part of us harms the whole of us, both individually and collectively.

We use the words wounded or broken spirit to refer to an injured or ill spirit. "Heart" is another word for "spirit." Some with a wounded spirit have been "cut to the heart." That which makes them alive has been injured. Some are injured in their spirit so profoundly that they never fully heal and return to their normal lives. Others are injured so severely that their spirit or heart is broken. When their injury is too severe to heal. They expire, spirit out. That which makes them alive is no longer there. They die.

Spiritual Healing Re-Visioned

When we are dysthumic, our spirit naturally works to become whole again. It works to heal and keep making us alive so we can fully recover, resume living a healthy life, and become what we are meant to become.

When either our body or mind is ill or injured, our spirit's inherent urge to keep living drives our healing. Our spirit itself is our urge to heal ourselves so that we may remain alive and become what we are meant to become. It drives us to heal the injuries and illnesses of our spiritbodymind and relationships with others. It drives us to help other's healing processes too.

In Thumotics, spiritual healing is re-visioned and clearly defined as the process of making whole again that which makes alive. Spiritual healing is a natural process that all living things do. We can observe the process at work. When anything living is ill or injured, it works to heal itself, keep living, and become what it is meant to become: a mature flower, tree, honey bee, cat, wolf, dog, crow, vulture, or human being.

Spiritual healing is not a medical, psychological, supernatural, religious, metaphysical, or psychic thing done to us. It is something we ourselves do. Our healing work is not something we choose to do. We just do it. More precisely, our spirit compels it.

However, there are times when our spirit cannot heal itself on its own. Sometimes we need help with our work of spiritual healing. Sometimes we need spiritual therapy.

Spiritual Therapy Re-Visioned as Thumotherapy

Having clearly defined spirit, spiritual, health, healing, therapy, and spiritual healing, we can clearly define spiritual therapy. It is therapy of, about, and related to that which makes alive, spirit.

The thumotic term for spiritual therapy is thumotherapy. As physical therapy is to the physical body, as psychotherapy is to the psyche, so thumotherapy is to the *thumos*, the spirit.

Thumotherapy is the process of attending to, serving, and taking care of another with dysthumia. Thumotherapists provide thumotherapy. They attend to what makes others alive, their spirit. They help those who cannot complete their spiritual healing on their own. They take care of those healing their spirit until they recover and return to their normal activities.

Thumotherapy differs from therapies for physical injuries and illnesses. It focuses on one's spirit rather than body.

While we can die from physical illnesses and injuries, we can also live relatively long lives with physical injury and illness. Many live relatively well with heart disease, diabetes, COPD, hypertension, amputations, and other illnesses and injuries.

Thumotherapy also differs from psychotherapy. It focuses on one's spirit rather than psyche. The spirit is quasi-physical. We feel it in the center of our chest, between our breasts, and behind our breast bone. The psyche or mind is non-physical but associated with the head and brain. Psychotherapists help with mental health and healing. Thumotherapists help with spiritual health and healing.

Rarely do we humans die of mental illness as the direct cause. Many live relatively well with depression, anxiety, bipolar disorder, schizophrenia, and other mental illnesses. However, we cannot live long or well when that which makes us alive is so ill or injured, that it cannot heal. We humans and other living things can and do die of broken spirits.

The Process of Thumotherapy

Since the spirit and its healing process is an organic, unfolding narrative, thumotherapy itself must be an organic, narrative process. It is the process of attending to, serving, and taking care of the narrative of the other's spirit and healing process. A thumotherapist joins, becomes a supporting character, and plays a role in the narrative of the other's spiritual healing.

Being a supporting character and playing a role in the other's spiritual healing maintains the thumotherapist's separate identity. It also assures that the healing work belongs not to the thumotherapist but the one in need of healing.

The role is to pay attention to, serve, and take care of the other's spiritual narrative of healing. The thumotherapist does not heal the other's spirit. With the attention, help, and care of the thumotherapist, the other's spirit heals itself. The thumotherapist attends to the other's spirit and its healing process, helps identify the needs and plan of healing, and takes care of the other as he or she heals.

The Beginning, Middle and End of the Thumotherapeutic Narrative

As any good story has a beginning, middle, and end, so does the narrative of thumotherapy. It begins with the thumotherapist facilitating his or her initial introduction into the other's spiritual narrative. Human thumotherapy begins with exchanging greetings and names, connecting spirit to spirit, and the thumotherapist expressing philothumy (love of spirit).

Once trust is established, the thumotherapist assesses the client's spirit, finds out what the client wants, what the client has done to fulfill his or her desire, what has happened in the process, collaborates to create a plan for healing, and helps the client initiate the plan.

In the middle of the therapeutic narrative, the thumotherapist attends to the client's progression or regression of healing, helps the client identify helpful and harmful consequences of actions, provides information, and explores with the client alternatives for future actions. He or she acknowledges, validates, and normalizes experiences, helps the client revise his or her plan of care, and cares for the client in his or her healing narrative.

The thumotherapeutic narrative reaches its turning point and begins to end when the client heals enough to return to his or her normal life. After this turning point thumotherapeutic contacts become less frequent and the thumotherapist prepares to exit the client's narrative. At their last meeting the thumotherapist and client reflect on their shared narrative, celebrate the client's healing, talk about what is ahead for the client, and that the client can return to thumotherapy if needed. They bid each other farewell and continue their lives.

The thumotherapeutic narrative might also end suddenly with the client's death when a client's spirit is so ill or injured that it cannot heal. Such a sudden ending could wound the thumotherapist's own spirit. Thumotherapists themselves need time for their own spiritual healing. Sometimes they need thumotherapy themselves.

When a thumotherapist needs thumotherapy, he or she does well to step out of the role of thumotherapist and simply be a human being who needs help with spiritual healing. It is best for thumotherapists to not identify themselves as thumotherapists but as those who provide thumotherapy. Thumotherapist is a role, not an identity.

From Spiritual Knowledge, Love, Healing, and Therapy to Spirituality

Having re-visioned and clearly defined spirit, spiritual, love of spirit, and spiritual knowledge, healing and therapy, we can now revision spirituality. Re-visioning spirituality is the topic of the next chapter.

8 SPIRITUALITY

*It is by being "natural" that one best recovers
from one's unnaturalness, from one's spirituality.
Friedrich Nietzsche*

Wondering About Spirituality

Wonder of wonders! We are alive rather than not, and we are alive together.

Spirit is that which makes us alive. Everything that is alive is a spiritual being because it has that which makes it alive, spirit.

Out of our love of life and being wondered by the mere fact of being alive, we are inspired to wonder about life and what makes us alive.

So far, in this brief introduction to Thumotics, we've wondered about what spirit is, loving care of spirit, knowledge of spirit, and spiritual healing. Now we turn our attention to wondering about spirituality.

Here is an interesting fact to be wondered by: The word "spirituality" is in the top ten percent of popular words right now. It is a very important word.

What is spirituality? To what does the word refer?

Begin with your own experience. What is spirituality to you? When you use the word, to what does it refer?

When you hear others say the word, what does it mean to them?

When you read "spirituality," what exactly does the writer mean? Does the writer define the word?

What is Spirituality?

As you wonder about spirituality, you might discover some of the same things I did. I discovered this:

First, I discovered that we often assume that we know what the word "spirituality" means. Speakers on the topic often do not define it. Neither do writers. They seem to assume that it means the same thing to everyone. Does it?

Barry M. Kinzbrunner, MD, co-author of *The Physician's Role in End of Life Care: A Practical Guide,* reported that a recent comprehensive review of clinical research articles on spiritual care found ninety-two different definitions of "spirituality" in the literature.

The lack of a general consensus among careful clinical researchers on the meaning of the word "spirituality" reflects the broader context of Western culture in which they work. We Westerners have no general consensus on what "spirituality" is.

For us Westerners, "spirituality" has a broad and varied range of meaning. Here is a short list of what it can mean-

1. Christian clergy
2. A person's process or experience of transcendence.
3. The quality or state of being dedicated to a god or goddess or Higher Power
4. A person's dedication to spiritual (immaterial, eternal) things rather than worldly (material, temporal) things
5. A sense of being connected with something bigger than oneself
6. Concern for meaning-making
7. Religious beliefs and practices in the context of an organized religion

8. Personal beliefs and practices apart from an organized religion; what makes one "spiritual rather than religious"
9. Personal beliefs and practices related to immaterial and eternal rather than material and temporal things
10. A personal, eclectic religion created by choosing beliefs and practices from various traditional religions, psychology, metaphysical, and self-help resources
11. A way of life informed by religious and/or existential beliefs and practices
12. Whatever one finds meaningful, whether it is associated with religion or not

Observations about Current Definitions of Spirituality

Note that none of the definitions listed above reflect a clear relationship to spirit. Rather than clearly relating to spirit, they relate to religious officials, religious beliefs and practices, and beliefs and practices related to existential philosophy and psychology.

More specifically, some of the definitions reflect the influence of Western monotheistic religions, especially Christianity. Those that do not overtly reflect the influence of Western monotheistic religions, reflect the more modern influence of existentialism.

They also reflect the influence of Enlightenment with its emphasis on rationality and assigning religious belief to the realm of private, personal opinion.

Dualism, the belief that there are two dimensions of reality, the physical and the so-called spiritual, and that the spiritual is more real and important than the physical, also influences some of the definitions.

The definitions are also anthropocentric in that they speak of spirituality only as it relates to human beings.

Other Important Perspectives on Spirituality

Some believe that since spirituality is so private and personal, individuals rightly define it for themselves. They believe there should be no general consensus on what the word means. Everyone should be free to have spirituality mean whatever they want it to mean to them personally. No one definition should be imposed on everyone.

Some believe that defining spirituality falsely limits, reduces, and puts it in a box. They believe words cannot contain spirituality. It is beyond words.

The beliefs that spirituality is something each individual defines or is beyond words, are themselves based on vague, unspoken definitions of spirituality: it means whatever one says it means to them. It is about something that is metaphysical and beyond words. Few things can be fully contained in or defined by words. Definitions are not the things they define. However, clearly defining things as best we can makes it possible for us to have coherent conversations about them, express our feelings about them, and learn more about them.

For others "spirituality" is how one escapes from the struggles of life. India is an excellent example of spirituality as escapism. Many see India as the most spiritual country on Earth. The people of India, like Buddhists, Christians, Muslims, Metaphysicalists, and others have a low view of life in this world. This world is not their home. They are just passing through. The sooner they return to their true home, the better.

For many in India the purpose of life is to escape reincarnation into this world of illusion, including the illusion of a self, and return one's true home beyond. The goal is to merge into Brahma, the supreme being, like a drop of water in the ocean. Indeed, we are "That" (Brahma) already.

They seek to escape from this world as much as possible while they are here. They do so by bathing in the Ganges, attending ceremonies in temples, practicing yoga, burning incense, praying to deities, chanting, singing, reading sacred writings, fasting, meditating, and engaging in other religious rituals.

All the while, India's social and environmental conditions are among the worst on our planet. Child mortality due to disease and starvation, stunted growth, and child brides are common. Women are gang-raped. Burning cow dung, crops, trees, and adulterated fuel pollutes the air. Over a billion gallons of raw sewage flow into the most holy Ganges River every day. All this and more in the most "spiritual" country in the world.

For still others, "spirituality" lacks any substantive meaning at all. Like "spiritual," as in "spiritual person," "spiritual beliefs," "spiritual place," "spiritual experience," and so on, "spirituality" just adds a "woo" quality to what they write or say. It helps sell books, holy water, crystals, jewelry, and other "spiritual things."

Problems with Spirituality

Imagine if each of the following words had over ninety different definitions:

Adversity
Authenticity
Biodiversity
Humanity
Majority
Mentality
Physicality
Sexuality
Sociality

What if we believed that the meanings of these words was private and personal, and each individual defined them for themselves?

What if we believed that defining these words put them in a box and falsely limited their meaning?

What if we believed they could not be defined, that words could not contain their meanings?

How could we have a conversation about them? How could we study and learn more about them? We couldn't.

How can we have a coherent conversation about spirituality when we have no general consensus on what the word means? When we merely assume we are talking about the same thing, how do we really know we are?

How can we study and learn more about it when we do not agree on what we are studying? Reliable, valid research on spirituality is impossible because researchers study at least ninety-two different things labeled "spirituality."

How can we practice it together when it means one thing to one and something different to another? How can we do it better, if we are not working to improve the same thing?

We lack a general consensus on what spirituality is because it is so closely related to both religion and psychology. Since we relegate religion to the realm of private and personal opinion, we relegate spirituality there too. We believe we have a basic human right to define our religiosity or spirituality however we want. Do we? Where did that belief come from?

Since we also conflate spirit with mind and fail to see it existing independently of the mind, we relegate spirituality to the domain of psychology, specifically existential psychology. In the domain of existential psychology, we conflate spirituality with the psychological process of meaning-making. It does not exist on its own apart from psychology.

We have serious problems with "spirituality." That "spirituality" is in the top ten percent of popular words makes our problem more poignant.

Re-Visioning Spirituality

In Thumotics, spirituality is re-visioned and clearly defined in the light of Homeric *thumos*. "Spirit" is a noun that refers to "that which makes alive." "Spiritual" is an adjective that means "of, about, or related to spirit." "Spirituality" is an abstract noun that refers to the quality of having spirit.

Spirituality is something we *have*. To have physicality is to have a physical body. To have mentality is to have a mind. To have sociality is to have social relationships. To have spirituality is to have spirit.

Spirituality is not restricted to humans. To have spirituality one must have spirit. One does not have to have a mind. As far as we know now, plants do not have a mind but they have spirit. One does not have to have a physical body to have spirituality. Goddesses and gods, assuming they exist, do not have physical bodies but they have spirit. All who have spirit and are therefore alive have spirituality.

As spirit exists in narrative form, so does spirituality. Spirit is the organic, dynamic, developing process of life. Spirituality is the organic, dynamic, developing narrative about spirit. Since we can see, hear, and feel our own and other's actions related to being alive, we can see, hear, and feel spirit. We can also record a spirit's actions in writings, photographs, sculptures, paintings, and audio and video recordings.

The narrative we tell about a living thing's actions related to spirit is its spirituality. It is the story of what a living thing does that promotes, protects, fulfills, harms, or ends its own life and the lives of others. It is an abstraction because it is not spirit itself. It is the narrative about spirit that we construct by pulling it out of the broader, whole, actual narrative of the lives of individual and collective living things.

In the broad, whole, actual narrative of life, spirituality is one subplot among the subplots of physicality, mentality, sociality, and many others. It is the subplot in which spirit is the main actor.

Spirituality is a narrative about something natural. It is part of the everyday narrative of life on this planet. It is not primarily about anything supernatural, religious, psychical, or metaphysical.

After we tell the story of a living thing's actions related to spirit, we can discuss, study, analyze, learn about, and influence it.

Not One, but Many Spiritualities

Since every living thing is a unique, one-time occurrence, every living thing has its own unique spirituality, its own unique narrative related to its own spirit and the spirits of others. No two spiritualities are the same narrative. Every spirituality is a unique blend of many characteristics.

We conclude well that there is no such thing as spirituality, only spiritualities.

Thumotic Spirituality

The specific type of spirituality introduced here is one re-visioned in terms of Homeric *thumos*. A thumotic spirituality is any spirituality that tells the story of a living thing's spirit within the parameters of the following seven characteristics:

1. Spirit is clearly defined in terms of Homeric *thumos*. Because it defines spirit in terms of *thumos*, it is-
2. Western- rooted, rather than Eastern turning
3. Nature-based rather than supernaturally based
4. Experientially-known rather than known by faith in an authority
5. Spirit-centered rather than belief, practice, or meaning-making centered
6. Presented in narrative form rather than static beliefs and practices
7. Life-affirming rather than life-denying

Three Intertwining Themes

Thumotic spirituality is an organic narrative of three intertwining themes: the descriptive, the evaluative, and the prescriptive.

The descriptive theme verbalizes the narrative of a living thing's spirit. It includes the life story, thumic norm, life-affirming desires, and the fulfilling of those desires.

The evaluative theme verbalizes the health and well-being of a living thing's spirit and its effectiveness in fulfilling its life-affirming desires.

The prescriptive theme verbalizes recommendations, based on the evaluative theme, for improving the health and effectiveness of the living thing's spirit.

Of utmost importance throughout the process of verbalizing the three intertwining themes of a living thing's spirituality is being mindful that no one's spirituality can be fully captured in words. Every verbal description is an abstraction from the real, living original. No verbal abstraction can possibly capture and express the full reality of a living thing's spirituality.

Difficulties

There are difficulties with re-visioning spirituality in the light of Homeric *thumos*. It requires revising our mental habits regarding spirituality. We do not do this easily or quickly. It can take decades to reach a general consensus on re-visioning spirit in terms of Homeric *thumos*.

Those most resistant to change are those who benefit from the status quo, especially those invested in materialism, scientism, religion, psychology, the medical industry, and profiting financially from the sale of related goods and services. Time will tell if we get there to not.

An added layer of difficulty comes with "spirituality" being both a live, organic, dynamic, developing aspect of a living thing and an abstraction. It is a human mental construct we create by the process of abstraction from the real, living thing that has spirituality.

From the broad, complete, living reality of one's life, we pull out and put into words its subplot about spirit. While our abstraction is based in the concrete reality of the living thing, it exists only in our minds and words. That spirituality exists as both a living, organic, dynamic, developing narrative of a living thing and a static abstraction in our minds and expressed in our words, adds complexity to our discussion of spirituality.

These difficulties and complexities can be identified but not fully addressed in this brief introduction. They will be addressed in future writings.

Spiritual Community

Community can support us in living more life-affirming lives. The next chapter begins with being wondered by the existence of spiritual communities and inspired to wonder about them.

9 SPIRITUAL COMMUNITY

*Without a sense of caring,
there can be no sense of community.
- Anthony J. D'Angelo*

Be Wondered

Wonder is the beginning of wisdom. Be wondered by the mere fact of being alive rather than not. Be wondered by the mere fact that we are alive together. We are not alone. We humans live with each other and all that is.

Every living thing is alive with and because of others. We all depend on each other for our lives. We humans depend not only on our parents but on all our ancestors for our lives. Without them we would not be alive. In a very real and natural sense, their spirit inspired our conception and birth and continues to inspire and keep us alive. Their spirit lives in us and makes us alive. We are spirited by their spirits.

If we have children, their lives depend on ours. Without us they would not be alive. Our spirits inspired their conception and birth and continue to inspire and keep them alive. Our spirits live in them and make them alive. They are spirited by our spirits.

We humans also depend on the spirits of the plants and animals we kill and eat. Their spirits, what makes them alive, make us alive. All of the plants and animals depend on the spirits of other plants and animals they consume.

All of us together depend not only on each other, but also on the earth, water, and air of our shared home, Planet Earth. Earth is our mother because we literally are of the earth and she sustains our lives. Our lives also depend on the Sun, Moon, and other planets in our solar system as well as all of the other stars and planets and forces in the rest of nature.

It is vital that we Westerners, now moving beyond our industrial economy, regain the wisdom many indigenous communities never ignored: we all are connected and rely on each other. We cannot deplete and pollute the earth, air, water, and the lives of those on whom we depend and expect to remain alive, healthy, and fulfill our purpose.

The previous chapter focused on how every living thing has a unique, once-occurring spirit and life. Everything has its own unique spirituality. This chapter shifts the focus from individuals to communities, specifically spiritual communities.

Community

We have a general consensus on the meaning of "community." A community is two or more individuals united by something they have in common. What they have in common could be their geographic location. They live in the same building, neighborhood, zip code, county, state, nation, hemisphere, planet, solar system, galaxy, or universe. It could be their species or racial or ethnic identity. It could be their gender identity or sexual orientation. Religious beliefs could be what community members have in common. Community members could also be united by a common cause or many other things they have in common.

Wondering about Spiritual Community

However, as discussed in Chapter Four, we do not have a general consensus on the meaning of "spiritual." As a result, we have no general consensus on the meaning of "spiritual community."

What is a spiritual community? What makes a spiritual community spiritual?

Current Definitions of Spiritual Community

Currently, "spiritual community" can refer to several different things. It can refer to a community of people who have the same or similar religious beliefs: A Christian church, Jewish synagogue, Muslim mosque, Buddhist sangha, Wiccan coven, or any other religious community.

"Spiritual community" can also refer to a community that shares a common practice or ritual like praying to a goddess or god, reading religious writings, meditation, yoga, tai chi, having a séance, reiki or other forms of alternative healing modalities, Tarot or other types of psychic readings, necromancy, spell work, nature walks, group therapy, education in religious ideas, or anything that members find meaningful to them.

"Spiritual community" can also refer to an other-worldly, supernatural, metaphysical community rather than a this-worldly, earthly, physical community. For example, some believe in a community of Ancestors, Elders, Saints, Ascended Masters, Angels, or other types of supernatural beings.

Since we have no general consensus on the word "spiritual", we have no general consensus on the meaning of "spiritual community."

Re-Visioning Spiritual Community

In Thumotics, "spiritual community" is re-visioned and clearly defined in the light of the Homeric word for spirit, *thumos*. The noun "spirit" is clearly defined as "that which makes alive." The adjective "spiritual" is clearly defined as "of, about, or related to spirit." So, "spiritual community" is clearly defined as "a group that is united together by being of, about, or related to that which makes alive, spirit."

Spiritual Characteristic

The members of a spiritual community can share in common a characteristic, interest, or practice that is of, about, or related to spirit. For example, a common characteristic all of us living things share is being spirited and, therefore, alive. The mere fact that we are spirited and alive rather than not unites us all together. The primary spiritual community is that of all living things.

This primary spiritual community is not exclusively human. Other animals are members of this primary spiritual community: rainbow trout, dolphin, turtles, squirrels, pigs, wolves, crows, vultures, hummingbirds, honey bees, butterflies, and dragonflies to name a few. Plants are members too: daffodils, violets, honeysuckle, azaleas, corn, wheat, mountain laurel, sourwood, and oaks.

There are also mixed-species spiritual communities. They live together in forests, valleys, plains, and seas and depend on each other to live.

Indeed, the community of all living beings is a mixed species spiritual community.

Spiritual Interest

Making and remaining alive is the ur-drive of spirit. It is the fundamental, primary common interest that unites all living things. The primary purpose of life is to live and live well.

All spirited beings are de facto members of the spiritual community that shares the common interest related to spirit, the common interest of remaining alive. All other communities are subdivisions of it.

Communities united by the common interest of remaining alive, work together to live and live well. They share in the common cause.

From a holistic perspective, the spiritual community of all spirited beings is greater than the sum of its parts. What affects one member of the community affects the whole community. What affects the community as a whole, affects all of its members.

Groups of individuals with conflicting interests join with each other by engaging in conflict. They are not a community; they are a disunity. They work against each other. They deny the ur-drive of spirit in themselves and others. They deny and harm their own spirits and lives and also those of all others.

Spiritual Practice

Members of a spiritual community can be united by engaging in the same practices that are related to that which makes alive.

Since many currently use the word "spiritual" for "religious", it is important to be clear that in Thumotics "spiritual" means "of, about, or related to spirit, that which makes alive." Spiritual practices are those related to spirit.

Mindfulness of Spirit

A basic spiritual practice implied by Thumotics is mindfulness of spirit. Spiritual mindfulness is a mental exercise that is related to spirit. It is the practice of focusing our mind on and giving our sustained attention to spirit. There are two forms of spiritual mindfulness: mindfulness of our own spirit and mindfulness of the spirits of others.

Mindfulness of our own spirit is the practice of focusing our mind on and giving our sustained attention to our own spirit. We do not have to buy anything to practice mindfulness of our own spirit. We do not have to wear special clothes or go anywhere special. It is not a self-help technique. It is not about trying to improve our spirit or change it in any way. It is simply being mindful of and paying attention to our own spirit.

As we practice mindfulness of our own spirit, our mind observes our spirit, becomes more aware of it, and retains information about it. We gain knowledge about and insight into our own spirit by practicing mindfulness of our own spirit.

Mindfulness of our own spirit is not a state we achieve and stay in. It is a practice. The practice is a process of focusing our mind on our spirit and returning our attention to our spirit whenever it shifts to something else.

There is no goal to be mindful of our own spirit for gradually longer periods of time. There is no goal to learn anything. The goal is to practice being mindful our own spirit. Some days we are better at it than others. It is that simple.

Mindfulness of the spirit of others is just as simple. It is the mental exercise of focusing our attention on the spirits of others. Their spirit is their aliveness. The spiritedness of each one we attend to is unique.

There is nothing to buy, nowhere special to go, and nothing to try to accomplish. The only goal to attain is to practice the process of being mindful of the spirits of others.

As we practice mindfulness of the spirits of others, we become more aware of their spirits, retain information about them, and learn more about them.

Mindfulness of spirit is the fundamental practice of philothumists, thumonauts, thumologists, and thumotherapists. It is one expression of spiritual love (love of that which makes alive). It is the source of spiritual knowledge, thumology. It guides the therapy provided by thumotherapists.

Mindfulness of spirit unites into a spiritual community all who practice it. When practitioners practice it together in each other's physical presence, their practice is strengthened.

Spiritual Care

A second spiritual practice, introduced in Chapter Five, on spiritual care, is caring for spirit. As with the spiritual practice of mindfulness of spirit, there are two forms of the practice of spiritual care: care of one's own spirit and care of the spirits of others.

Care of one's own spirit, autophilothumy, is the practice of relating to our own spirit in ways that help rather than harm it. When practicing autophilothumy, we do what affirms rather than denies our own spirit and therefore, our own life.

Basic autophilothumy practices include eating safe, fresh, nutritious food; drinking fresh water; breathing fresh air, working to fulfill our purpose, resting, sleeping, playing, enjoying pleasure, protecting ourselves from danger, being with others who love and care for us, and avoiding those who do not.

In Thumotics, self-denial is a spirit-denying, life-denying practice to be avoided except in extreme circumstances where we die protecting ourselves or others we care for.

Care of the spirits of others, allophilothumy, is the practice of relating to others in ways that help rather than harm them. When practicing allophilothumy we affirm rather than deny the spirits and lives of others.

Some of the basic practices of allophilothumy include allowing others to live their lives and fulfill their unique purposes, helping others fulfill their purpose, helping others heal when they are ill or injured, humility, joining in creative and life-affirming work together, and playing together.

Killing to Live

As mentioned earlier in this brief introduction, we kill to live. We cannot not kill and live. We humans are not the only spirited ones who grieve when another living thing is killed. Others grieve too.

Since we affirm spirit and life and have to kill other animals and plants to in order to live, we do well to kill only when necessary for us to live. We do well to kill reluctantly and as respectfully as we can, and with sorrow. There is no joy in killing others. Only those with disordered spirits and minds take joy in killing others.

We show respect to those we kill to live by killing them as quickly and painlessly as possible. We show respect by wasting nothing of the one we kill, but using all of the one we kill to affirm life.

Indigenous groups who have not been infected by life-denying Western ways and practice spiritual care, including life-affirming killing, remain a resource to us Westerners finding our way forward out of the aftermath of the Industrial Revolution.

Spiritual care unites those who practice it into a spiritual community. Those who practice it in each other's physical presence, gain strength in their practice by doing so.

Conclusion

As more of us humans form communities based on shared spiritual characteristics, interests, and the two simple practices of spiritual mindfulness and spiritual care, we will make life-affirming differences for ourselves and all others with whom we share life.

The Afterword that follows asks those of us who care about revising the narrative of life on this planet, to do two things.

AFTERWORD

This brief introduction is only a beginning. It is the beginning of a new, public conversation about our sense of wonder, life, spirit, language about spirit, loving care of spirit, spiritual knowledge, spiritual healing, and spiritual community.

We humans cohabit this planet with all other spirited things. Everyone who cares about spirit as re-visioned in this brief introduction has an essential role to play in the narrative of our life together. We all have our own experiences to share of being wondered by life. We all have spirits with life-affirming desires to fulfill. We all have new habits to develop regarding how we talk about spirit. We all have much to learn about caring for the spirits of those with whom we interact.

We need some playing award-winning roles as philothumists, thumonauts, thumologists, thumotherapists, and thumogogues of individuals and thumotic communities.

Imagine the story of life on this planet and how it would change with more of us being wondered by the mere fact of being alive, fulfilling our spirit's life-affirming desires, caring for our own spirit and the spirits of others, learning more about spirit and how to heal it as well as how to form and sustain healthy spiritual communities. How does your spirit respond when you imagine that world?

If your spirit responds with a "Yes!" to that world, then please do two things:

1. Share this book with others you know who might also care.
2. Contact me through my website, www.MarkWNeville.com

Thank you for taking these steps now so that together we are taking action to fulfill our spirits' life-affirming desires.

Mark W. Neville

FOR FURTHER READING

Primary Sources

Homer. *The Iliad*. Various translations.

Homer. *The Odyssey*. Various translations.

Secondary Sources

Brann, Eva. 2008. *Feeling Our Feelings*. Philadelphia.

Bremmer, Jan. 1983. *The Early Greek Concept of the Soul*. Princeton.

Caswell, Caroline P. 1990. *A Study of Thumos in Early Greek Epic*. Leiden.

Crites, Stephen. 1971. *The Narrative Quality of Experience*, Journal of The American Academy of Religion, vol. XXXIX, no. 3, pp. 291-311.

Cunliffe, Richard John. 1963. *A Lexicon of the Homeric Dialect*. Oklahoma.

Green, Christopher D. and Philip R. Groff. 2003. *Early Psychological Thought: Ancient Accounts of Mind and Soul*. Westport.

Koziak, Barbara. 2000. *Retrieving Political Emotion: Thumos, Aristotle, and Gender*. Pennsylvania.

Mayeroff, Milton. 1971. *On Caring*. New York.

Padel, Ruth. 1992. *In and Out of the Mind: Greek Images of the Tragic Self*. Princeton.

Snell, Bruno. 1982. *The Discovery of the Mind in Greek Philosophy and Literature*. Dover.

Sullivan, Shirley. 1999. *Sophocles' Use of Psychological Terminology*: Old and New. Carleton.

Mark W. Neville

A THUMOTIC LEXICON

-A-

Allophilothumia: loving care of the spirits of others.

Animism: the view, not that everything has a soul (*psyche*), but that everything has spirit and is alive.

Anti-spirituality: any spirituality that denies rather than affirms spirit and life.

Ascension: the attempt to rise up beyond one's ego and this world in order to identify with an imagined higher being that is one's true self; a life-denying practice based on a low view of humanity, life, and nature.

Aspire: to spirit toward. When we aspire to something our spirit rather than our body or mind drives us there.

Asthenothumia: weak-spiritedness.

Athumia: non-spiritedness; a neutral condition of spirit; one of the three general categories of spirit-related conditions, the other two being dysthumia and euthumia.

Autophilothumy: loving care of one's own spirit.

-B-

Becoming: the process of constant change of everything that exists.

Being: an imaginary state of unchanging existence.

Body: from our human perspective, the physical aspect of spirited beings, that which appears to be relatively solid to us.

Bradythumia: slow-spiritedness.

Broken spirit: see clastothumia.

-C-

Clastothumia: broken-spiritedness; a condition of spirit, frequently fatal, in which our spirit is so damaged and overwhelmed and we lose our desire or ability to remain alive.

Conspire: to spirit together. Those who conspire to do something, join their spirits together to do it.

Cryothumia: cold-spiritedness, "ice in the veins."

Cyclothumia: cycling spirit; cycling through recurring conditions of spirit; for example, phases of hypothumia and hyperthumia.

-D-

Death wish: the desire to die, a symptom of a weak, sick, wounded, or broken spirit.

Dethumia: negated-spiritedness, the condition after one's spirit is denied, diminished, or otherwise negated.

Dethumize: to deny, diminish or otherwise negate spirit.

Dispirit: to not spirit, to take away spirit, deny spirit. To dispirit another is to deny and diminish their life and what makes them alive. To be dispirited is to suffer having one's spirit and life diminished and denied.

Disthumia: diffused-spiritedness; the condition of a dissipated, ungathered, unfocused, scattered spirit.

Doing: used in contrast to "being" to refer to living. There is no state of just being. To live is to do and become.

Dynathumia: strong-spiritedness; seen in those, for example, who survive significant challenges, crises, and ordeals. Resilience is an expression of dynathumia.

Dysthumia: ill- or troubled-spiritedness; one of the three general categories of spirit-related conditions, the other two being euthumia and athumia.

-E-

Eastern turn: the adoption of Asian religious beliefs and practices by Westerners.

Ego: self; we humans do not have egos, we are egos. We are ourselves. The clearer we are about who we are, how we are both unique and similar to others, what our natural abilities are, and living from our ego, the more we affirm our life and the lives of others, the healthier we are.

Eirenothumia: peaceful-spiritedness.

Endothumotic: internally-spirited.

Engagement: the opposite of ascending and transcending; the process of fully living in and of this world.

Erotothumia: erotic-spiritedness; a condition of spirit that features sexuality.

Esprit de corps: the spirit of a group; the experience of a group sharing a common spirit that is more than the spirits of the individuals that comprise the group.

Eternal life: endless life; we do not know that life is inherently eternal. We do know that life is contingent on the living reproducing and sustaining themselves. Life is potentially eternal. It is also potentially temporary.

Euthumia: well-spiritedness; a healthy, whole condition of spirit; one of the three general categories of spirit-related conditions; the other two being athumia and dysthumia.

Exothumotic: externally-spirited.

Expire: to spirit out. When spirit exits any living thing, it dies.

Extrothumia: outwardly directed spiritedness.

-F-

Fellarothumia: sucking-spirit, drains the life (spirit) out of others. "She sucks the life right out of me." "Just being with him makes me tired."

-G-

Glycothumia: sweet-spiritedness, either authentic or feigned, expressed, for example, in a soft tone of voice, with a smile, and kind words and deeds.

Gratitude: the pleasure felt when a desire or need that one cannot gratify for oneself is gratified by another.

Gratify: to fulfill another's desire or need that the other is unable to fulfill alone.

-H-

Hadrothumia: thick-spiritedness.

Hyperthumia: high-spiritedness.

Hypothumia: low-spiritedness.

-I-

Introthumia: inwardly oriented spiritedness.

Inward turn: intentionally closing our eyes and turning our attention away from engaged living in the world and inward to our thoughts and emotions; can be either therapeutic or self-indulgent escapism.

Inspire: to spirit in. When we inspire another, we increase their spiritedness.

-J-

-K-

-L-

Liberthumia: free-spiritedness; the condition of living according to one's own ways and outside dominant social norms. A liberthumiac's non-conformity is driven by her spirit rather than her body or mind.

Life-affirming: that which says yes to life and promotes and celebrates it.

Life-denying: that which says no to life and weakens, tames, or ends it.

-M-

Malthumia: mean-spiritedness.

Megathumia: great spiritedness, palpable presence, wide-spread, historical influence.

Melanothumia: dark spiritedness.

Mind: the cognitive function of spirited beings.

Minded: having cognitive ability, conscious, aware of self and others.

Mindedness: the state or process of being minded.

Mindfulness: the practice or state of intentionally using the mind to attend to something.

Misothumia: hatred of spirit, life, and living.

Morothumia: dull-spiritedness.

-N-

Nature: everything that exists. From the perspective of Thumotics, nothing is supernatural, beyond nature.

-O-

-P-

Personal religion: an individual's personal collection of beliefs and practices picked from various religions.

Philothumia: loving-spiritedness.

Photothumia: light-spirited.

Preparedness: having the skills and resources to sustain one's live in extreme conditions.

Pyknothumia: dense, contracted spiritedness.

Pyrothumia: fiery-spiritedness.

-Q-

Quasi-physical: near, almost, as if physical. Ancient Greeks considered *thumos* to be quasi-physical, located in the chest, behind the breast bone, and associated with the thymus gland.

-R-

Religion: a set of beliefs about existence and how to live that were created by someone else to which one seeks to conform.

Respirate: to spirit again. Respiration occurs when spirit returns after it left. Fainting and resuscitation are examples of respirated.

Responsibility: able to respond.

Responsible for: able to respond on behalf of another.

Responsible to: able to respond to others.

-S-

Schizothumia: split-spiritedness.

Siccothumia: dry-spiritedness.

Soul: another word for mind, psyche, personality, and perspective.

Spirit: that which makes alive.

Spirit-related: about or associated with that which makes alive.

Spirit-related intelligence: understanding of and the ability to regulate one's spirit.

Spirit of place: the animating aspect of an area of land, a building, or any other place that makes the place unique.

Spirited: the state of having spirit, alive.

Spiritedness: aliveness, the state of being spirited.

Spiritual: of, about, or related to spirit (*thumos*).

Spiritual being: a living being whose primary identifying characteristic is its spirit rather than its body or mind; for example, if great-spiritedness is the primary identifying characteristic of a woman, she is a spiritual being.

Spiritual beliefs: beliefs about spirit (*thumos*), not religious or metaphysical beliefs.

Spiritual discipline: the training of one's spirit (*thumos*) by spiritual practices and exercises in order to improve its condition.

Spiritual exercises: activities that test or increase one's control of spirit (*thumos*); a spiritual exercise can be done one time whereas spiritual practices are exercises done on a regular, ongoing basis.

Spiritual experience: an experience of one's own or another's spirit (*thumos*).

Spiritual growth: the maturing process in living a spirit-centered life.

Spiritual guidance: the act of guiding another's spirit to a more life-affirming life.

Spiritual journey: the process of becoming more adept at caring for one's own spirit and that of others.

Spiritual life: a life devoted to taking good care of one's own spirit and that of others.

Spiritual person: someone adept at taking good care of their own spirit and that of others.

Spiritual practices: activities done on a regular basis that exercise one's spirit.

Spirituality: the condition of having spirit. As physicality is the condition of having a physical body, mentality is the condition of having a mind, and sociality is the condition of having social relationships, so spirituality is the condition of having spirit.

Stenothumia: constricted-spiritedness.

Survival skills: skills that enable one to stay alive in life-threatening circumstances.

-T-

Tachythumia: fast-spiritedness.

Thauma: Ancient Greek word for wonder.

Thermothumia: warm-spiritedness.

Three great mysteries: life, sex, and death.

Thumogogy: spiritual guidance, leading another's spirit from one mode of being to another.

Thumonaut: an explorer of spirit.

Thumos: The Homeric Greek word for spirit, that which makes alive.

Thumotherapy: attending to, serving, taking care of spirit so that it may heal.

Thumology: the scientific study and knowledge of *thumos*, spirit.

Thumotic spirituality: the condition of having spirit defined in the light of *thumos*. The narrative of one's spirit and life.

Thumotics: the science, therapy, and spirituality of spirit.

Thyme: an herb the Ancient Greeks associated with *thumos*, spirit.

Thymus: a gland the Ancient Greeks associated with *thumos*, spirit.

Toxothumia: toxic-spiritedness.

Tramotothumia: wounded-spiritedness.

Transformation: used in contrast to transcendence to refer to the ongoing process of change living beings experience through the course of their lives.

Transcendence: seeking to rise beyond life in this world into an imagined eternal realm of being; a form of escapism.

Transpire: to spirit through. The story of a life, or any part of it, is the story of what transpired; What transpired is the story of what a spirited one lived through and how. The story of an entire life, of what transpired, is not just a story. It is the story of a spirit.

-U-

-V-

-W-

Wonder: a semi-euphoric state of attending to a person, place, thing or activity that evokes marvel and curiosity.

Work: activities the living do to continue living: obtaining food, water, and protection (shelter and clothing) and becoming what they are meant to become.

Wounded spirit: the weakened condition of a spirit harmed by another.

-X-

-Y-

-Z-

Mark W. Neville

ABOUT THE AUTHOR

Mark W. Neville, M.Div. is the author of the innovative and inspiring *Your Spirit, Your Life* series. He has over thirty years of training and experience caring for individuals and families as a counselor, educator, writer, and thought-leader specializing in spiritual care.

For ten years he worked with one of the premier hospice and palliative care organizations in the U.S. providing patient and family care; teaching healthcare providers of all disciplines about spiritual care, bereavement, and leadership; developing best clinical practices; leading multidisciplinary clinical teams, and designing innovative programs.

He now has a private practice near Asheville, North Carolina where he lives with the love of his life, Lisa. They love life, especially trees.

CONTACT THE AUTHOR

www.markwneville.com

www.facebook.com/MarkWNevilleMDiv

www.ingramcontent.com/pod-product-compliance
Lightning Source LLC
Chambersburg PA
CBHW071822200526
45169CB00018B/587